THE NURSE CONSULTANT'S HANDBOOK

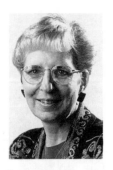

Belinda E. Puetz, PhD, RN, currently is President/ CEO of Puetz & Associates, Inc., in Pensacola, Florida. Dr. Puetz serves as editor of four nursing journals, manages five national nursing specialty organizations, consults in continuing education and staff development, and teaches continuing education activities for nurses.

Dr. Puetz received a diploma in nursing from the Henry Ford Hospital School of Nursing in Detroit, and a baccalaureate in nursing from Indiana University in Indianapolis. Her master's and doctoral degrees in adult education were granted by Indiana University in Bloomington.

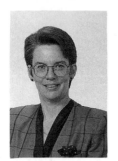

Linda J. Shinn, MBA, RN, CAE, is currently Senior Vice President and Principal, Consensus Management Group (CMG) in Washington, D.C. CMG is a consulting firm specializing in providing services to trade and professional associations and charitable and philanthropic groups. Ms. Shinn was previously the Deputy Executive Director and Chief Operating Officer of the American Nurses Association.

Ms. Shinn received a diploma in nursing from the Memorial Hospital School of Nursing in South Bend, Indiana, and a baccalaureate in political science from Indiana University. Her master's in business administration was granted by Indiana Central University. She received an honorary doctorate from the University of Indianapolis in 1994.

THE NURSE CONSULTANT'S HANDBOOK

Belinda Puetz
Linda J. Shinn

SPRINGER PUBLISHING COMPANY

Springer Publishing Company, Inc.
536 Broadway
New York, NY 10012-3955

Cover design by: Margaret Dunin
Production Editor: Susan Gamer

97 98 99 00 01 / 5 4 3 2 1

Library of Congress Cataloging-in-Publication Data

Puetz, Belinda E.
    The nurse consultant's handbook / Belinda Puetz, Linda J. Shinn.
        p.   cm.
    Includes bibliographical references and index.
    ISBN 0-8261-9520-2
    1. Nursing consultants—Vocational guidance.   I. Shinn, Linda J.
II. Title.
    [DNLM: 1. Specialties, Nursing.   2. Consultants.   3. Professional
Practice.   4. Entrepreneurship.   WY 90 P977n 1997]
    RT86.4.P84   1997
    610.73—dc21
    DNLM/DLC
    for Library of Congress   96-47041
                                                                        CIP

Printed in the United States of America

To my mother, Elizabeth Puetz,
the first entrepreneur in the family.

B.E.P.

To Dorothy and Richard K. Shinn, my first consultants, for their advice,
counsel, love, and support. To Richard G. Shinn, my current consultant,
for his spirit, sense of humor, and perseverance.

L.J.S.

Contents

Foreword

In these chaotic times it is often difficult to work out just where change is leading us. With the radical shift in the focus of health care and the dramatic changes required as a response to economic constraints, jobs are disappearing and roles are shifting faster than anyone can cope with. The real challenge of the time is to be able to see past the changes themselves and to interpret their meaning within a broader context of the global shifts affecting everyone and every aspect of life. The chaos is simply a sign of the drama and the intensity associated with the transformation from a manufacturing age to an information society.

New roles are emerging in nursing too. The old "bed"-related hospital-based roles for nursing are diminishing quickly, and the opportunity to provide nursing service in a different context and a new environment is unfolding faster than there are nurses to fill the emerging roles. The "noise" of the transition can be heard in the reactions from nurses in a variety of settings, who are seeing the loss of old roles but are not yet able to "see" the new roles beckoning those who are astute enough to respond. This is always the paradox of transformation; those who are stuck in mourning for experiences that are quickly passing often are not prepared to engage the opportunities that are unfolding. Indeed, there are many who see in those opportunities such loss of what they know that they oppose them vigorously, all in the name of "protecting" what is quickly passing.

It is somewhere between these two views of reality that the role of the consultant finds its value. The consultant is much like a guru with experience. Consultants see change far enough in advance of its impact that they can help give both form and meaning to it. They are the agents of the winds of change. While consultants may take many roles and operate at various levels of expertise, they have at least one thing in common—their adaptability to change and their ability to engage it directly. They are often bellwethers of change, and they often model direct response, exhibiting a level of energy that results from a convergence of opportunity and action.

What is, perhaps, most surprising is how little regard there really is for the role of consultant, especially in nursing. Often the consultant is over-looked as a professional colleague: undervalued as a nurse, because of her or his perceived distance from the patient; and underappreciated as a con-sultant, because so many nurses really don't understand who consultants are or what they do. Successful consultants are especially suspect, because they often reflect an image of economic and personal independence that is considered an anomaly in many nursing circles. Furthermore, it often appears that no one really wants a consultant around—unless there is a real need for a consultant, evidenced by an inability to "take care of things on our own" or to "use our own resources."

The truth is, however, that the consultant is as important and vital as any other member of the health care team. Although the role of consultant often falls outside of the circle of the work team, it is just as valuable as any other pursuit in the interest of good health service. The consultant's greatest asset is *not* being part of the circle of work, *not* operating inside it, and *not* seeing work and relationships from the same perspective as those directly involved. An external frame of reference, altered insights, and a fresh viewpoint are gifts the consultant brings to the table, along with genuine skill, knowledge, and experience. Thus the consultant offers a rich mix of value that will both enhance and advance the enterprise.

The dark side of the role, if there is one, is that the good, ethical con-sultants belong to no one, own nothing and take nothing away when they have expended their value. Consultants must slip away as quietly as they began and leave behind the only real thing they have to offer of any value: knowledge and how to apply it. Consultants must also realize that they serve the organization and that when they are done, they must leave every-thing behind in the ownership and control of the people in the organiza-tion. Satisfaction, for the consultant, must come from the reward that is reflected in the success of other people's actions and the outcomes of the application of their work—gained, in part, through the interventions of the consultant.

Not everyone can be a successful consultant. There is probably no role which invites so many people to it and then proceeds to eliminate them quickly. Clearly, it is not for the faint of heart or mind. It takes great strength to handle the role of "outsider"; to "leave behind" whatever hap-pened in the workplace; and, for many in the role, to accept the long hours of travel and isolation. It takes great skill to engage people in a process or activity that they might most want to avoid. Continual attention to enhanc-ing knowledge and refining skills will be necessary to keep the consultant informed and able. The hours are variable; the time is everyone else's; and the demand for creativity and intensity is sometimes overwhelming. Good theatrics (presentation is very important), enthusiasm, (especially when there is no reason for it) and an absolutely impenetrable spirit are essential to longevity in the role.

Also, the science and method of consulting are important in sustaining the role. It takes a real understanding of the consulting process, and of the elements it comprises, to be successful in the role. Much has been developed with regard to what works and what doesn't, as this book amply testifies. The words in this text will assist both the neophyte and expert in broadening their understanding of methods and processes which facilitate the successful exercise of the role. Increasing both knowledge and skill in the consulting process benefits both consultant and client.

The authors have put together in this text a full view of the role of the consultant. What they have prepared for the interested reader is a breadth of understanding about what the role entails and what it takes to be a successful consultant. What adds to the credibility of this book is the fact that both authors are successful consultants themselves: They have "been there," and they are bringing their own experience to this work. The flow of this book—from defining what consultation is, through the consulting process to the needs of the business—helps the reader understand the many facets of building a successful consultant practice.

Of special importance in this text are the business aspects of building relationships, markets, and services. What nurses bring to the consulting role does not always transfer to managing the business. The chapters on business issues, marketing, and networking are important aspects of the consulting practice that should be of real value to the reader.

The book ends with an important chapter regarding the personal needs and characteristics of the consultant in her or his role. The need to be personally disposed to the role is vital to any consideration of building a consulting practice. From the organization of one's files to the management of time, this chapter helps the potential (or current) consultant get an idea of personal issues affecting the building of an effective consulting practice. As the authors point out, the ability to manage and discipline choices, activities, and time is a vital prerequisite for successful entrepreneurs.

There has probably never been a better time than today for the role of the consultant. The unending value of change alone provides a foundation for consultation. Indeed, there is more work in the field than there are competent consultants to undertake it. The need for new insights, skills, formats, processes, innovations, and creativity continues to grow as society reinvents itself within a new paradigm. While it is certainly tough "out there," it is also exciting and challenging. As the authors clearly outline in their chapter on legal and ethical considerations, there is much to be aware of—and cautious of—as contracts and conflicts are dealt with in the consultant's practice. With the right blend of savvy, skill, knowledge, and attitude, however, there is more than enough opportunity for the person with the right blend of talent, entrepreneurial spirit, and enthusiasm. The challenge to share in creating the future in a host of different ways is unparalleled in history. Regardless of specific aptitudes, there is more than enough work to do and more than enough places that are demanding the skills of a good consultant.

In this book, Belinda Puetz and Linda Shinn offer their colleagues a rich resource for developing the role of the consultant in any setting. Nurses interested in this wonderful career will find much within these pages to answer their questions and stimulate their interest. Taking the reader from interest to constructing a consulting practice,—in practical and straightforward prose,—this book is a definitive tool that can help answer almost any question anyone might have about the business of consultation.

It is my hope that the arena of the nursing consultant will expand and grow in acceptance, respect, and contributions within the greater nursing community over the next several decades. It is to that end this book most vigorously contributes.

TIM PORTER-O'GRADY, EdD, PhD, FAAN
Senior Partner
Tim Porter-O'Grady, Inc.
Atlanta, Georgia

Preface

The idea for this book was conceived at a time when jobs for nurses were plentiful and hospitals appeared to be the mainstay for the delivery of health care. Consideration was being given to intrapreneurial roles for nurses within institutions, and a few free spirits, unafraid of risk and confident of reward, moved into the ranks of consulting.

This book was envisioned as an addition to the sparse literature about the nurse consultant as well as an update of those readings already on the shelf. Also, the authors were curious about how the practice and business of consulting in nursing had changed since Sister Mary Jean Flaherty's study of nurse consultants was published 10 years ago.

In a decade, the world has turned upside down. Nurses are being laid off and are having to acquire skills in new types of practice and work in ever-changing venues. Hospitals are merging, closing, or affiliating with bigger chains or venturing into new lines of business. Businesses, including those in the health care industry, are outsourcing a number of their services or hiring temporary personnel or agencies to do jobs once done by employees. Technology too is changing the way nurses work, learn, communicate with colleagues, conduct research, provide care, and do the business of their professional organizations. The aging of the profession, (many of its members are baby-boomers), is resulting in greater personal reflection and more inquiry into what to do with the rest of one's professional life, overlaid with the need to pay more attention to family and community. All of this has set the stage for nurses to turn to the consulting role in ever greater numbers.

This handbook for nurse consultants is dedicated not only to our families but to all our colleagues confronting the vagaries of the world of work and wondering, "Do I have what it takes to be a consultant?" It was written to provide insights into the realm of consulting, to offer tips on starting or fine-tuning a consulting practice, and to describe the world of today's nurse consultants.

Special thanks to Sister Mary Jean Flaherty, PhD, RN, Dean, The Catholic University of America School of Nursing, for permission to replicate the study of nurse consultants. The results of our update of this study are integrated throughout the book. A bouquet of appreciation to those nurse consultants who responded to the questionnaire providing insights, answers, questions, and food for thought for this nurse consultant's handbook. And to Patricia Adkison our gratitude for her help with the nurse consultant's survey and many other details that resulted in the publication of this book.

BELINDA E. PUETZ
LINDA J. SHINN

1

What Is Consultation?

Consultation is, quite simply, providing advice to others. The advice might be in the form of guidance, information, knowledge, expertise, or solutions. Some people view consultants as problem identifiers and problem solvers. Others look to consultants for options in responding to issues and dilemmas. "Consultants can provide a series of options that they know have been successful in similar situations. They also can recognize what potential solutions are not likely to work well" (Furlow, 1995, p. 13). More and more consultants are being called on to serve as an "extra pair of hands" to accomplish a project or task that an organization does not have the internal resources to handle.

Consultation can be short term or long term, free or for a fee, focused on process or content, and provided by recognized authorities external to a group or experts within an organization. Advisers are used in all walks of life—at work, at play, at home, in the school, in the religious congregation, in the hospital, and the nurse-run clinic or physician's office.

Cohen (1991) defines consulting as giving advice or performing services for others in return for compensation. He further suggests that regardless of one's area of interest or expertise, becoming a consultant is possible as one's special interest, unique experience, or expertise is demanded somewhere in the marketplace. Lange (1987) calls consulting a helping, task-oriented process based on meeting client's needs. Helping or consulting is a natural role for nurses who are focused on meeting the needs of people. This book is addressed primarily to the nurse as consultant and was written to help those who are considering a consulting practice. In this text, consultation is also considered as an activity performed on a regular basis and managed as a business.

The business environment of the 1990s is fertile territory for consultants. As organizations decrease the number of workers on the payroll, replacement of employee talent often comes in the form of consultation as organizations outsource tasks, projects, or functions. Outside problem solvers are also used to supplement employees' aptitudes or to increase a company's competitive edge. Consultants are frequently called on for their training skills; for new ideas; as a neutral, disinterested party to offer another opinion or options; or for expertise needed by an organization only occasionally. Consultants also may be engaged because a funding source or regulatory body has insisted on it (Harris, 1995).

Eras of uncertainty and rapid change of pace are also fertile times for consultants as people in businesses look for insights, ideas, or answers to perplexing issues or try to determine what to do next. "When uncertainty abounds, consulting flourishes as people seek out experts to 'show them the way'" (Furlow, 1995, p. 13).

Consultants are usually specialists in a specific practice or business area. Just as nurses specialize in gerontology, occupational health, oncology, or dermatology, consultants are experts in major business venues, such as strategic planning, human resources, malpractice law, or health care finance. Nurse consultants can be found in publishing, continuing education, accreditation, and a variety of clinical practice areas.

The giant strides in technology have resulted in vast new consulting opportunities. For example, nurses are specializing in the management of information and consulting with health care institutions on record management, building customized databases, or manipulating computer software programs that trace critical pathways.

Consultants might specialize by business line, such as hospitals, home care agencies, hospices, or associations. Consultants often work in a particular geographic locale, such as at a local, regional, state, or national level. Consultants may concentrate in the public or private sector. International consulting is an avenue opening to many, particularly in business and health care. Trade and professional journals are full of advice about moving into international venues. The World Bank, the Federal government, and several trade and professional associations are financing consulting activities abroad.

Consultants may practice full-time or "moonlight" as a consultant while holding a full-time job. Consultants work as sole proprietors, in partnerships, in think tanks, or as employees of large corporations.

The New Jersey–based Consultants Bureau estimates that there are more than 100,000 independent consultants in the United States and 70,000 management-consulting firms. The bureau estimates that $18 to $20 billion a year is spent for consultation in the public and private sectors ("Odd Jobs," 1995). Industry experts predict that there will be double-digit growth rates in the practice of consulting over the next 5 years (Byrne, 1994).

People losing jobs are joining the consultant ranks in growing numbers. Employers are releasing employees from their payroll only to hire the same people back as consultants, primarily to save on personnel benefit dollars. Those in midcareer often turn to consulting as a way to gain a measure of independence and control of their own destiny. Still others supplement their incomes through consulting. Retirees are taking the edge off boredom, keeping mentally and physically agile, or sharing a lifetime of experience by joining the consulting ranks. Nurses too are moving into the consulting ranks in ever increasing numbers.

HISTORY OF CONSULTING

History is replete with examples of humans seeking advice. In ancient times, oracles, wise people, and gods were consulted with regularity. In modern times, experts are sought for advice on everything from making war to making money.

Han Fei Tzu, adviser and founder of a Chinese school of philosophy, is regarded as the first consultant in recorded history. Machiavelli is regarded as the first management consultant in the Western world (Hay, 1988).

The accounting industry is frequently thought of as among the early business consultants. External, independent, third-party financial audits have been the order of the day in business for years. These third-party observers have carved out a niche in reviewing and commenting on the process of receiving, keeping track of, and spending money. The results of such review and comment are critical to the well-being of proprietary enterprises that must provide operational results to stockholders and to nonprofit organizations that rely on contributors or members for survival. Today, the "big six" accounting firms not only provide advice on finance and budget, but also have expanded their practices to include other aspects of business such as staffing, marketing, production, and sales. Some even have a health care practice. Several employ registered nurses.

In many respects, the profession of nursing from its inception has been a practice of consultation. Much of the caring that has constituted the practice of nursing since the early days included advice to patients and others. The counsel frequently took the form of guidance on wound care; information on communicable diseases, such as tuberculosis; and expertise in ministering to the patient with tetanus or the baby with colic.

The entrepreneurial approach to consultation has been the traditional approach. An entrepreneur, employed external to an organization, was invited into an organization to provide tips on problems or issues of the day. The entrepreneur was frequently selected on a competitive basis not only for expertise but also for price. In health care, early consultants in the form of engineers provided counsel on work processes and conducted time-and-motion studies of nurses providing patient care.

The late 1980s witnessed the advent of the internal nurse consultant and intrapreneurial consultant. Internal and intrapreneurial consultants arose in health care, particularly in nursing, as people were called to move from unit to unit or facility to facility within a complex of organizations to provide expertise or to generate new ideas or approaches to problems. For example, the clinical nurse specialist has frequently been called upon to provide practice consultation across clinical units or specialties. Clinical nurse specialists often provide advice to other nurses or care partners on treatment modalities, interventions, standards, or techniques. "Intrapreneurship offers nurses new opportunities to harness their creative energies—and reap the rewards—without having to start a business or give up the financial security of employment" (Manion, 1994, p. 38).

However, Block (1981) notes that the challenges of the internal consultant are: organizational politics to overcome, bosses to satisfy, company goals to achieve, processes or hierarchies to follow, and financial control procedures to work through. Such challenges can lead the consultant to tell half-truths in an effort to spare feelings and please the boss. The hazards posed for the internal consultant include being "shot" as the messenger of bad news and being viewed by colleagues as the good or bad guy or gal or a snitch. Because of status or rank, the internal consultant may not have access to high-level people in an organization, or to key vendors or external consultants. The internal adviser may suffer from anxiety about the job if the outcome of the consultation does not produce the anticipated results. Bosses might apply pressure for specific recommendations or preferred end products.

At the same time, there are advantages to consulting from within an organization. The advantages include a knowledge base: familiarity with the organization; with its goals, processes, and key players; and with the company's strengths and weaknesses. The internal consultant might accomplish an assignment more quickly than an external consultant who must spend time learning about the organization and its people. In addition, the internal consultant is often around to see the outcomes of the consultation and can help fine-tune end results or make necessary midcourse corrections. An external consultant does not often have the satisfaction of knowing what happened as a result of advice given. The internal consultant is often readily available and can be freed up quickly to take on a consulting assignment. The company is spared a time-consuming search for an external adviser. The company knows the quality of the work of the internal consultant and saves time that might be spent on checking the references and past work products of an external consultant.

Other nurses as consultants are those who are expert witnesses in a court of law. This is an example of the nurse providing expertise in a community venue. Hospice nurses or home health nurses who provide advice to the ill or dying at home are yet other exemplars.

Nurse consultants have had traditional roles in providing guidance to schools of nursing to assist them in meeting accreditation standards and preparing for site visits of such organizations as the National League for Nursing. Nurse staff development or continuing educators have provided counsel to those preparing for accreditation by the American Nurses Credentialing Center or approval by a state nurses association of their continuing education activities. Nurse executives have often reached out to colleagues in nursing administration to act as coaches and confidants in preparing for an accreditation visit by the Joint Commission on Accreditation of Healthcare Organizations.

Public health nurses were among the first nurse consultants. They visited homes, schools, offices, and community centers to provide counsel, care, and curative measures to the poor, uneducated, and infirm. Gradually, state boards of health and departments of public instruction began hiring nurses to serve as advisers across communities on matters from record keeping to communicable diseases. Nurses serving in the military can also be included in the early consulting ranks, because they advised corpsmen on caring for others, conferred with generals and admirals on health practices, and counseled scores of battle-weary combatants on grief and loss. Nurse researchers have expanded their practice from the school or laboratory to the clinical site providing advice to patients, care providers, families, and communities. They are serving as advisers and collaborators with clinicians to unearth, describe, and test new knowledge.

CONSULTATION IN NURSING

This book is an exploration of consultation in nursing. It is a quest for the *who, what, where, when,* and *how* of that aspect of nursing practice known as consultation. A profile of the nurse consultant was first gathered and published in 1989 by Flaherty and Demoya, who looked at aspects of the consultation practice and demographic variables of consultants. The authors of this book have expanded on Flaherty and DeMoya's inquiry nearly 10 years later.

In mid-1995, we conducted a survey of nurse consultants based, in part, on Flaherty and DeMoya's earlier survey (1989). The original form was adapted with Flaherty and DeMoya's permission. We conducted a pilot test of the survey. Forty-four surveys were mailed for the pilot test; 2 were returned as undeliverable; and 23 were filled out and returned—a 52% return rate. Of the 23, 2 have discontinued their consultation, 1 retired, 1 decided her services were not consultation, and 1 critiqued the survey tool rather than answer the questions posed. Eighteen ($n = 44$; 41%) completed the survey.

Changes were made in the survey form as a result of the pilot test. The survey was then mailed to 356 nurse consultants whose names were obtained from the "Directory of Nurse Consultants" published in the *Journal of Nursing Administration.* Of these, 141 surveys were returned, for a return rate of 40%; 128 of the surveys, or 36%, were usable.

Today's nurse consultants practice in a wide variety of settings and 46% of the respondents report working as a consultant part-time. Most of the respondents (75 of 128; 59%) reported being in practice by themselves. Almost all got started on their own initiative; most state they have spent 5 to 15 years in the consulting business. In addition, the preponderance of nurse consultants are between the ages of 40 and 55. Almost all of those responding to the question regarding gender were female (96 of 128; 75%) and some (14 of 128; 11%) were male. All but six respondents reported being educated at the master's level or above. One reported the associate degree as the highest degree held. Most respondents were married, and more than half reported having no dependents.

The results of this survey of nurse consultants are woven throughout the book. The findings describe the nurse consultant, the types of consultation nurses provide, preparation for the consulting role, hours worked, challenges and choices encountered, and the economics of consulting. In some instances, comparisons with the earlier data are provided.

This book also reflects much of the knowledge of the authors, who have more than 20 years of combined experience in consultation in the nursing, health care, business, and association communities. Most important, this book is a "consultation in progress" for those readers thinking about new ways of living and working, enhancing consulting practices, acquiring new knowledge and skills, or giving the benefit of their knowledge and expertise to those in the marketplace.

CONSULTANT ROLES

A consultant is one who provides expertise or helps meet someone else's needs. The consultant can assume the roles of coach, motivator, mentor, teacher, facilitator, confidant, sounding board, change agent, fact finder, expert, observer, or counselor. Care must be taken to distinguish the consulting role from the role of manager. Block (1981) states: "A consultant is a person in a position to have some influence over an individual, a group, or an organization, but who has no direct power to make changes or implement programs. A manager is someone who has direct control over the action. The moment you take direct control, you are acting as a manager" (p. 1).

Coach, Motivator, Mentor, and Teacher

In these roles, a consultant might work with a client who has a basic body of knowledge or a basic set of skills, and needs to amplify or practice what is known. Alternatively, the client might need to change a set of behaviors. Enter the consultant who can augment knowledge or skills; supervise practice; encourage positive behaviors or identify strategies for behavioral changes; stimulate thinking about matters from a different vantage point; foster creativity or a new way of looking at the world; provide expertise, information, wisdom, or enlightenment; or strengthen fledgling efforts.

Facilitator, Confidant, Counselor, and Sounding Board

Often the consultant is a purveyor of encouragement or a silent partner who listens and offers observations or options for a different way of doing things. The consultant may serve as the "keeper of the process" so that the client can focus on substantive issues or content with staff or customers. The consultant may serve as a testing or proving ground for new ideas or new ways of handling familiar projects or issues. The consultant might be a recipient of frustration or anger or a receiver of confidences that cannot be shared elsewhere.

Change Agent, Expert, Observer, and Fact Finder

The consultant can be a provider of new or controversial ideas or a lightning rod for introduction of change or a new order of things. The consultant can bring aptitude, ability, or vision to a setting. As observer or fact finder, the consultant might detect or discover errors in information, thinking, or processes; uncover behaviors or skills previously untapped; or identify deficiencies creating barriers to progress. The consultant might also bring new knowledge or facts to a situation.

FRAMEWORKS OF CONSULTATION

There are two frameworks for consultation: process and expert (Berger, Ray, & DelTogno-Armanasco, 1993). Process consultation usually involves working closely with an organization's staff to identify problems, develop options for resolving the problems, and select and implement the best solution. The consultant usually serves as a guide or sounding board. An organization's staff remains an integral part of the process throughout and decides on strategies and solutions to deal with the matter at hand. A good example of process consultation is strategic planning. The consultant might provide the framework for the planning process, serve as the planning facilitator, and design the planning document once the planning work is done. The clients (or staff) are an integral part of the entire planning process, from creating a mission to making assumptions to setting goals and identifying the actions that must be taken to implement the goals. The consultant serves only as an escort; the organization's leaders are in the driver's seat, making the necessary turns and corrections to position the institution.

Content consultation, conversely, relies on a body of knowledge, customized information, or special expertise to help an organization work with an issue. This type of consultation is often referred to as expert consultation. It differs from process consultation in that the consultant involves the organization's staff minimally, if at all, and solves the problem or decides which solution is best to fix the problem. For example, an authority on violence in the workplace or sexual harassment provides education on how to identify and deal with these two workplace problems.

As an aside, the authors of this book are uneasy with any kind of consultation wherein an organization's staff is minimally involved. We contend that a consultant cannot be helpful to any party unless it "buys in" and is involved. Take the earlier example of a consultant providing education on workplace violence. The consultant might speak to a dutifully gathered group of employees and emphasize how to deal with violent patients only to learn from the question-and-answer period or from evaluations of the presentation that the issues of concern centered on violence between and among employees. In this example, an assessment of employees' needs would have gone far to enhance the consultant's effectiveness in providing content consultation. A consultant cannot fix a situation and expect it to stay fixed without the investment of the client in the repair. Successful consulting is a two-way street involving a mix of the consultant's skills and the client's needs, with both participating thoroughly in the process.

PROCESS OF CONSULTATION

Steps in the Process

The process of consultation will be addressed in more detail in chapter 2, but nurses should remember that consultation is akin to the nursing process, which involves assessment, planning, implementation, and evaluation.

First, the consultant assesses the situation. For example, in a consultation project where the consultant seeks to assist a national nursing organization in obtaining accreditation of its continuing education program from the American Nurses Credentialing Center (ANCC), the nurse consultant conducts a site visit to the client and there reviews the ANCC criteria with the client while determining the extent to which the client's program currently meets these criteria.

The second step, "planning," occurs during the initial site visit, when the nurse consultant and the client together determine what needs to be done for the program to meet the criteria. For example, perhaps the client and consultant plan that biographical data on speakers as well as information on the sessions they present at the annual convention will henceforth be collected on ANCC prescribed forms.

The third step in the process is "implementation." In this step, the plans identified by the nurse consultant are carried out by the client.

The fourth step, "evaluation," may consist of another site visit by the nurse consultant, who then determines the extent to which the plans have been accomplished and the extent to which the program now corresponds with the ANCC criteria.

To repeat: the consultation process includes assessment, planning, implementation, and evaluation.

Skills

The skills needed to perform consultation activities parallel those of nurses wishing to implement the nursing process in their daily work. The skills that are needed to establish a successful consulting practice are the following (Metzger, 1993, pp. 7–16):

Diagnostic ability
Problem-solving skills
Specialized knowledge
Communication skills
Marketing abilities
Business sense

Personal traits might also be listed here (as they are in Metzger, 1973), but we prefer to treat them as a separate topic (see below, page 12).

Diagnostic Ability. Like the nurse entering a patient's room and assessing the patient, the nurse consultant must be able to assess or diagnose the problem being presented. Often the problem is obscured by several factors that are not immediately apparent to the consultant. As with a patient who focuses on one symptom or set of symptoms (such as a distressing cough) to the exclusion of the larger problem (the patient smokes nearly two packs of cigarettes daily), the client may home in on the symptoms of the problem (e.g., a "difficult" patient) rather than on underlying factors (enabling behaviors of the staff that contribute to the patient's behavior or cause the patient to be difficult). In all cases, the nurse consultant must remain objective about the problem, whether it is a patient or a dysfunctional system.

The consultant also must remember that he or she will view the problem from a perspective formed by his or her educational and experiential background. That is, an evaluation consultant will view situations as requiring some assessment of their worth or value; a communications consultant will define the problem as one of communication. The consultant must avoid this tendency to view situations narrowly by being aware of it and by attempting to approach all consultation situations with a "worldview," bringing in individuals with perspectives other than the consultant's when indicated. For example, the nurse consultant engaged to assess the effectiveness of a staff development department might subcontract with an individual with expertise in compensation if the compensation of the staff in the department is in question.

The nurse consultant must recognize in all instances that the ability to diagnose accurately is a key to being able to perform the next steps of the process. If the problem is not defined correctly, then the solutions will not be identified correctly. The nurse consultant must have the ability to analyze situations with a critical eye.

Problem Solving.   The nurse consultant must be able to identify ways to solve the problems identified. This is not always as simple as defining the problem, developing solutions, and communicating them to the client. In the example above of the patient with a cough, changing behavior to avoid the symptoms may require more behavior modification than the patient desires to undertake. The patient may not want to quit smoking just to get rid of an annoying cough. Sometimes, the consultant has to solve the problem in small steps the client is willing to take, such as switching to a cigarette with lower tar and nicotine.

The consultant's objective, outsider's view is used here to provide a perspective that the client has not known before. For example, the nurse consultant working with staff and a "difficult" patient may identify behaviors of the staff that reinforce some of the difficult behavior of which the staff is complaining. The nurse consultant then points out those behaviors—tactfully, of course—and the staff members gain an insight that they may have not before considered.

Because the nurse consultant's suggestions may be threatening to the client, particularly when they involve changing long-standing behavior patterns, the consultant must be tactful and considerate in presenting these ideas. The nurse consultant also must be able to help the client change the behaviors that are necessary to solve the problems.

Specialized Knowledge. The nurse consultant must possess specialized knowledge—that knowledge is why consultants are engaged by clients. The more specialized the knowledge, however, the more limited the market for that knowledge. A nurse consultant who has specialized knowledge about how associations run will be more in demand than an individual who knows only about writing a newsletter or managing an information system.

The specialized knowledge also must be current knowledge. Futurists predict that the knowledge base will soon turn over every 12 to 18 months. Clients do not want outdated or obsolete knowledge applied to their problems or used to meet their needs. Critical to the nurse consultant's survival will be the ability to stay up to date, amass new knowledge, and apply the knowledge to consultation assignments.

Nor do clients want consultants who cannot apply their knowledge to the client's particular situation. A theoretical approach to a client's problem may not be as helpful as a practical solution that can be easily implemented. In addition, clients do not want a "boilerplate" response to dealing with their particular situation. The successful consultant will not try to make "one size fit all" but will bring a customized approach based on specialized knowledge made applicable to the client's unique circumstances.

Communications Skills. It is vitally important for the nurse consultant to be able to communicate clearly in both written and oral forms. Perhaps the most important communication skill, however, is listening. The nurse consultant must be able to hear what the client is saying to diagnose the problem correctly. Mentally racing ahead to solutions while the client is talking about the problem may lead to fixing the wrong problem. The nurse consultant must be skilled in interviewing individuals—asking questions that elicit the desired information, probing where there appear to be gaps, and summarizing and reflecting back the essence of the conversation.

The consultant must be an expert in writing and presentation skills. Writing skills are necessary in preparing proposals and reports. The nurse consultant must be prepared to present proposals to potential clients, persuading them to engage his or her services. The nurse consultant must be ready to provide a clear report of findings and recommendations arising from the consultation (see chapter 2). Consultants also may be expected to present the findings of their consultation projects to decision makers; in these instances, the consultant must be skilled in persuading the client to accept, or at least listen to, the consultant's view of the situation. The results of the consultation are usually conveyed in writing and orally. The power of the written and spoken word may hold the key to influencing the client to make the necessary changes to solve the existing problems. In these presentations, the consultant must have great facility with the data gathered—and the ability to recount the findings and recommendations in his or her report and respond to comments and questions about methodology, observations, findings, and recommendations. The consultant must also be able to produce and use audiovisual aids to help in presenting findings and recommendations (see chapter 6).

Marketing Acumen.   Nurse consultants must be able to market their unique services. If no one knows what consultants can do, no one will hire them. In marketing services, consultants use communication methods to convince potential clients that they are the best persons to address the client's particular situation. Many nurses are confident of their skills in practice; they possess the necessary expertise to serve as consultants, but they are less comfortable with selling their services. These nurses do not realize that they are marketing their services successfully all the time: when they respond to the challenging patient, when they address the concerns of the family, or when they suggest a change to the department head. These examples, however, are not as difficult as marketing consultation skills—selling oneself as the product or service. Selling oneself takes lots of effort. Marketing is a key to the success of a consultant (see chapter 6).

Business Sense.   In addition to specialized knowledge, the consultant must know how to run a business. Consultants may be sole proprietors of their own business, partners in a business, or part of a larger corporate structure. In any case, knowledge about all aspects of a business—from legalities to accounting to negotiating contracts for products and services or client agreements to record keeping—are crucial to the consultant's well-being (see chapter 5).

PERSONAL TRAITS OF CONSULTANTS

There is a common set of personal characteristics consultants must have irrespective of the role they play. These attributes are listening, observation, objectivity, flexibility, patience, persistence, self-confidence, humility, and integrity. These traits, by the way, are as important to building and maintaining a consulting practice as they are to working with clients.

Listening

Statistics suggest people hear about 25% of what is being said. A consultant who hears only 25% of what is said will not last long in the business. Covey

(1989) propounds that most people listen to respond rather than to understand. A good habit, then, is to listen to understand rather than to respond. There are no better skills for a consultant to have than those of listening. In the survey of nurse consultants we conducted in mid-1995, the ability to "listen" was the one piece of advice several respondents (5 of 107; 5%) listed as good advice for those just beginning in the consulting business.

Observation

A good test of your powers of observation is to put this book down and cover the face of your wristwatch with your hand. Now describe the watch face to a friend, a colleague, or your spouse. No doubt, the description was not 100% accurate. The message is clear—people often do not see things that are right before them. (Even nurses, who are taught to observe, observe, observe, frequently fail this exercise.) The ability to notice all that is going on around an individual—the nuances, body language, raised eyebrows, messy desk, spotless bookcase, sagging draperies, books on the coffee table, or wear on a computer keypad—is paramount to the consultant.

Objectivity

Being fair, unbiased, and impartial is an attribute a consultant must acquire and maintain. Objectivity requires a consultant to gather all data, listen to a variety of viewpoints, observe the obvious and obscure, question until full understanding is achieved, and remain open-minded and willing to explore options.

Flexibility

In today's world, there is no one right way to do anything. Agility in thinking a matter through, willingness to consider a variety of viewpoints, and versatility in problem resolution are a necessary part of the consultant's armamentarium. A close cousin to flexibility is creativity—another important skill for the successful consultant. Creativity might be looking at things from a different angle, or applying aspects of music, drama, art, or literature, or a totally different discipline to working through an issue.

Patience

Poise, composure, and equanimity in the face of conflict, error, uncertainty, and an ever-changing client base and ever-changing clients' needs are important tools to include in the consultant's kit. Patience is as important to the consultant's own self-preservation as it is to working with customers.

Persistence

Endurance, stamina, and tenacity are ingredients consultants must bring to assignments as well. The ability to "stick with it" has helped many a consultant through difficult times in generating business and in working with clients to be clear about problems and anticipated outcomes.

Self-Confidence

Being certain about one's own skills and abilities is a necessary precursor to taking on a client assignment. Confidence also requires the ability to know "what is not known," and to acknowledge when the consultant does not have the knowledge or skills to take on an assignment or a part of an assignment. Confidence also requires being able to "stick to your guns" in the face of challenge or adversity.

Humility

Humility is a natural partner to confidence. Modesty and temperance in approaching and working with clients fosters a give-and-take that can result in an effective use of the consultant as a resource and growth on the part of clients. The consultant who thinks he or she knows everything and can learn nothing from a client or colleague is in the wrong business. Conversely, a consultant must have enough ego to deal with a great deal of ambiguity, uncertainty, and risk.

Integrity

A commitment to honesty, fairness, and a code of ethical conduct is a critical component of a consultant's makeup. The exercise of prudence and goodness in dealings with others is an important skill to bring to the consultant's practice.

Special attention to the roles and skills of consultants will be addressed throughout this book. Equally important are the ethical challenges faced by consultants, which are addressed in chapter 8.

IS CONSULTING FOR YOU?

At the dawn of the 21st century, there are nurse consultants in such diverse areas as association management, human resources, durable medical equipment, quality, productivity improvement, mergers, acquisitions, telecommunications, insurance, and marketing. Nurse consultants have emerged in such industries as pharmaceuticals, insurance, law, technology, tele-communications, architecture, landscaping, public relations, and publishing. A cadre of nurse advisors work for such agencies as the World Health Organization and the U.S. Department of Health and Human Services. As noted previously, the "big six" accounting firms have added nurses to their consultant rosters, as have several Fortune 500 companies and private foundations. Nurses have come forth as political advisers, consultants to those who hold public office, or officeholders themselves who then advise on health and public policy.

Many people, in all walks of life, are tempted to go into consulting today. The vagaries of the health care marketplace and uncertainties in hospitals, schools of nursing, and industry make the idea of consulting attractive to nurses. One of the questions asked in the survey of nurse consultants we conducted was: "If you could offer a novice consultant some advice, what would that advice be?" Several respondents urged those thinking about entering the consulting field to think carefully before stepping into the role, as consulting is not for everybody. Although there are many aspects of consulting that seem ideal, such as greater freedom and flexibility in designing work schedules or working from one's home, there are extraordinary challenges in the life of a consultant as well. Self-discipline, marketing one's expertise, rejection, loneliness, and erratic cash flow are some of the hazards those new to the consulting business often find overwhelming or difficult to overcome. One survey respondent suggested working with an experienced consultant, free, as a good strategy to determine if an individual likes the business. Another aid is thoughtful, careful completion of the Nurse Consultant's Checklist in Table 1.1. Still another is the questionnaire in Table 1.2, on areas of interest and expertise.

Lange (1987, p. 191) suggests that a consultant must first know himself or herself and reports that the following characteristics are associated with successful consultants:

1. Need for achievement, commitment to excellence, and desire to be a winner
2. Commitment to the task, energy, stick-to-it attitude, and willingness to assume responsibility
3. Aggressive ability to take on realistic tasks; preference for moderate risk, but not for gambling
4. Alertness to opportunities, and speed in seizing and converting them to advantage
5. Objective, realistic, unsentimental, and businesslike approach to solving problems
6. Sense of stimulation when given feedback on performance
7. Self-confidence and optimism in novel situations

TABLE 1.1   Nurse Consultant's Checklist

So you want to be a consultant—circle the answers that best describe you.

1. I am a self-starter.	Y	N
2. I like working by myself.	Y	N
3. I have good listening skills.	Y	N
4. I am good at selling ideas.	Y	N
5. I am good at marketing my skills and talents.	Y	N
6. Although I am bothered by rejection, I learn from the experience and move ahead.	Y	N
7. I am good at keeping confidences.	Y	N
8. I rarely lose my "cool."	Y	N
9. I am creative and generate lots of ideas.	Y	N
10. I love to work.	Y	N

Note. If you answered yes to all of these questions, consulting may be for you.
If you answered no to one or more, think carefully about moving into the consulting role.

TABLE 1.2   Identification of Areas of Expertise or Interest

Identify areas of expertise or interest by completing the following inquiries:

1. List the practice areas in which you excel.
2. List the special credentials or certification you hold.
3. What are the hobbies or pursuits you find yourself drawn to repeatedly?
4. In what areas have people told you that you excel? Are these the same areas about which people regularly seek your advice?
5. What are the problems you like to solve?
6. If you could have any career or profession you choose, what would that be?

Note. Review the answers to the preceding questions. Are there common themes or issues that emerge? These themes may identify areas of expertise or interest around which you might build a consulting practice.

8. Valuation of money as a measure of success more than for wealth itself
9. Active managerial style, future orientation, organizational skills
10. Outstanding communication and social skills
11. Sensitivity and receptiveness; ability to analyze people quickly

Achievement, Excellence, and Winning

Today's consultant succeeds with a commitment to excellence in the consulting practice, which manifests itself in a reputation for high-quality work. Helping others leads to a sense of accomplishment, which cannot occur without a desire to outdo the competition.

Commitment, Energy, Stick-to-It Attitude, and Responsibility

Consulting has peaks and valleys—such as wondering where the next client is coming from or worrying about whether the product provided for a client truly meets the client's needs. These peaks and valleys demand an ability to stay with it and stay level. There is no one to stand over a consultant's shoulder, prodding him or her to meet a deadline. The consultant has to start and keep going on his or her own initiative. The consultant has to do what he or she promises, being solely responsible. Good health is another part of this equation, particularly the harnessing of energy and stamina, and conveying an impression of well-being.

Ability to Take Risks Yet Not Go Too Far

A consultant must be willing to introduce new ideas or a new order of things, perhaps venturing into untested waters without sacrificing the quality of a product or one's own reputation. The consultant must be able to balance danger with certainty.

Desire to Seize an Opportunity

A consultant must be on the lookout constantly for new client opportunities, constantly marketing himself or herself in all that is said and done. The consultant must be ever alert for new ideas, new ways of doing things, and for levers and bridges that might lead to new connections or venues for work or unique approaches to client's problems.

Businesslike Approach

Consulting is a pursuit that demands evenness in temperament, attitude, and demeanor. Consulting necessitates a sense of humor and the ability to laugh at oneself. It requires the ability to balance achievement and winning with rejection and loss—of a client or an opportunity. Consulting demands the ability to look at all sides of an issue and put personal biases, no matter how compelling, aside.

Feedback on Performance

In many respects, the consultant must be his or her own critic or evaluator, assessing "how am I doing," through feedback from clients, repeat business, or referrals by clients to other assignments.

Self-Confidence

Consulting requires surefootedness in all work undertaken; it is not for the faint of heart. It requires ease and grace in admitting or saying, "I don't know." Consulting provides ample opportunity to plow new ground by threading knowledge and expertise into a new set of skills to take on the unusual or the uncommon or to blaze new ground. Self-confidence requires balancing ego with a bit of humbleness.

Money

Cohen (1991) suggests that consultants can make six-figure incomes. Large international consulting firms make millions of dollars in fees every year. Every dollar comes through high-quality work, excellent reputation, energy, and enterprise. In the survey of nurse consultants conducted by the authors in mid-1995, of those who responded to a question regarding annual income, 23% (23 of 99) reported an annual net income of less than $5,000; 23% (23 of 99) reported earning more than $60,000 annually; 12% (12 of 99) reported earning $ 75,000 to $100,000 annually.

Organization and Future Orientation

Order in one's work and work habits provides the leverage and time to market one's services, gain new knowledge and skills, and identify trends and opportunities embodied in those trends. As a consultant, planning ahead for a project, and a work day, getting new clients, and completing a client assignment can make all the difference between succeeding and becoming an also-ran.

Communication and Social Skills

Will Rogers said, "I joked about every prominent man in my lifetime, but I never met one I didn't like" (Kaplan, 1992, p. 638). Although the consultant does not have to like everyone he or she meets in consulting, it is necessary to have the social graces, dexterity, and common sense to deal with a variety of different people. Communication and social skills can help the consultant sell his or her product or advice in almost any setting. Excellence in communication skills helps the consultant build a reputation. Proficiency in communication can also assist in persuading a prospective client to pay the consultant's fees.

Quick Study

In consulting, sizing up people or situations accurately and quickly is a must. The inability or failure to do so can result in missed opportunities, misunderstandings, and misadventures. The ability to make a decision is paramount, and the consultant rarely has the luxury of deciding when to decide.

Change

The authors would add one additional characteristic to Lange's list—the ability to deal with continuous change. The 21st-century consultant will be challenged repeatedly not only to help clients deal with change but also to deal with constant variations in the practice of consulting. Astounding advances in knowledge and technology will open new ways of doing business. For example, a few consultants are assisting clients in making decisions through the use of groupware technology—an electronic decision-making tool that permits people to evaluate and test options anonymously, build a common vision, set priorities, and aggregate and evaluate decisions. Technology will provide new avenues for getting business; for example, consultants are beginning to woo clients via the Internet.

If the reader is uneasy about any of these 12 characteristics, consulting may not be the job of choice. Remember, too, that change usually occurs in the presence of a precipitating event, such as an environmental disaster, health hazard, or business downturn. A precipitating event, such as loss of a job, or a fight with a boss or colleague, should not be the impetus to get into consulting. Make sure to arrive at the decision to enter consulting after careful consideration of the pros and cons, and a complete understanding of what is required in running a business, marketing products and services, accounting for income and expenses, and complying with applicable law.

It is important for an aspiring consultant to know clearly whether or not he or she has enough financial reserves or resources to call on while getting a consulting practice started or getting established as a consultant in an already constituted practice. As a rule of thumb, figure on 3 to 5 years to get established as a consultant. Before starting a consulting business, look for a coach, mentor, or role model to smooth the way or to provide an opportunity to learn about the business. Be sure family members are supportive of the nurse consultant working at home, toiling for long hours, and interrupting holidays or vacations for those assignments that must be taken on while getting started in the consulting business.

If the reader has determined that consulting is for him or her, there are many helpers and helpmates. Hundreds of books and articles have been written on the subject of consulting; several appear in the references for this book. Scores of associations provide information, resources, advocacy, and consultant networks. These associations include the Association of Management Consultants, the Institute of Management Consultants, and the Society of Professional Business Consultants. Consulting associations by practice specialty, such as the Association of Fashion and Image Consultants or the American Association of Healthcare Consultants, exist. Some professional associations have a consultants' section or consultants' directory, for example, the American Industrial Hygiene Association.

The Association of Management Consulting Firms publishes a career kit designed to help those seeking a career in management consulting. The association also offers a course on management consultation and a directory of consultants.

There is even a certification program for consultants. Certified Management Consultant (CMC) is a designation attesting to surviving the rigors of the consulting business for at least a 3- to 5-year period, holding a baccalaureate or the educational equivalent, work experience, professional activity, adherence to the consultant's code of ethics, client references, and an interview by a team of CMCs. The Institute of Management Consultants (IMC) offers the CMC. IMC also publishes a Code of Ethics to guide the consultant in ethics and integrity. The authors hope this book will be of assistance to the reader who is thinking of becoming either an internal consultant or an entrepreneur. The practical tips contained in this book may start the reader on the consulting road or may result in a renewed commitment to the nurse's current career path.

SUMMARY

Consulting—providing advice to others—is becoming a popular career choice for today's job seekers and a popular next step for job holders, including nurses. Whether the consultant is an entrepreneur or institutionally based, his or her skills must include an ability to be objective, to listen, to communicate, to solve problems, and to market. At the same time, the consultant must keep abreast of rapidly expanding knowledge and the gigantic leaps in technology, and be comfortable with change. There are a myriad of resources for the emerging consultant and for those who have been in the business for a long time.

For those readers who are nurse consultants, we trust the insights and advice of the authors will be helpful and the experience of others in the business insightful. Perhaps the reader will pick up a new tip to help in generating new business, finding new prospects, or developing a new skill to add to the consultant's toolbox. For those nursing students who pick up the book or who are required to read parts of it, we anticipate that the student will find excitement and caution, and, perhaps, a career avenue he or she had not considered. The student will also find this book full of information that may help with that next paper or class presentation. This book should also be of value to those readers who may need to retain a consultant. A look behind the scenes at what makes a consultant tick, what is ethical consulting practice, how a consultant's business might be structured and fees established, what goes into a contract for consultant services, and how a consultant markets products or services can be valuable assets for the potential client or customer.

For all who pick up this book: Welcome, and read on.

REFERENCES

Berger, M. C., Ray, L. N., & Del Togno-Armanasco, V. (1993). The effective use of consultants. *Journal of Nursing Administration, 23,* 65.

Block, P. (1981). *Flawless consulting.* San Diego: Pfeiffer & Co.

Byrne, J. A. (1994, July 28). The craze for consultants. *Business Week,* p. 61.

Cohen, W. A. (1991). *How to make it big as a consultant* (2nd ed.). New York: AMACOM.

Covey, S. R. (1989). *The seven habits of highly effective people.* New York: Simon & Schuster.

Flaherty, M. J., Sr., & DeMoya, D. (1989). An entrepreneurial role for the nurse consultant. *Nursing & Health Care, 10,* 5, 259–263.

Furlow, L. (1995). So what good are consultants anyway? *Journal of Nursing Administration, 25,* 13–15.

Harris, M. (1995). Consultants: An administrator's viewpoint. *Journal of Nursing Administration, 25,* 12–14.

Hay, P. (1988). *The book of business anecdotes.* New York: Facts on File Publications.

Kaplan, J. (1992). *Bartlett's familiar quotations.* Boston, MA: Little, Brown & Co.

Lange, F. C. (1987). *The nurse as an individual, group or community consultant.* Norwalk, CT: Appleton-Century-Crofts.

Manion, J. (1994). The nurse intrapreneur how to innovate from within. *American Journal of Nursing, 94,* 38.

Metzger, R. O. (1993). *Developing a consulting practice.* Newbury Park, CA: Sage.

Odd jobs. (1995, January 8). *Washington Post,* p. H–4.

2

The Consultation Process

As pointed out in chapter 1, consultation is a process not unlike the nursing process, involving distinctly different activities in phases, stages, or steps that result in a unified, productive, and effective whole. Understanding the process of consulting with its attendant policies, procedures, and techniques helps the nurse consultant obtain and maintain the necessary skills to function efficiently and effectively in the consulting role.

Using the nursing process as the framework for the consulting process has two advantages. First, the nursing process is a model with which nurses are already familiar; second, it provides a structure through which the nurse consultant can function in providing services to the client. The steps in the nursing process correspond to the stages or phases of the consulting process. Activities occurring during consultation can be clustered within the steps of the nursing process: assessment or diagnosis (which includes negotiating), planning, intervention or implementation, and evaluation.

ASSESSMENT OR DIAGNOSIS

Assessment is the first step in the process. In this step, the client and nurse assess each other; the problem in the situation; and possible solutions to the problem; they also negotiate certain aspects of the consultation project, such as cost, time frame, and individual responsibilities. At this initial stage, the nurse consultant begins the process of selling consultant services. Persuading someone to engage a nurse consultant is as important for the internal nurse consultant as for the consultant who is in the consulting business and, thus, external to the organization.

An inquiry about consultation services usually begins with either a telephone call or a written request for a proposal. The client contact is critical. It is a "foot in the door" and must be handled as a sales opportunity and an occasion to get as much information about the consulting assignment as possible.

Telephone Requests

A potential client calls and asks for information about the consultant's services and the cost. On some occasions, the prospective customer has identified an external consultant and merely seeks additional information about fees in order to make the case with a manager or a board that an array of consultants have been contacted and two or three price quotations obtained. The nurse consultant might readily identify such an inquiry when the caller asks about fees during the early portion of the conversation rather than inquiring about the consultant's skills for pursuing a particular assignment. One of the authors has had a caller state that he was comparison shopping.

Although is tempting to brush off such inquiries, take the time to query the caller about the goals of the consultation and to obtain information about the prospective client. Always follow up on an inquiry, provide a proposal if required, and send information about the consulting services and fee structure. This is a way of advertising the nurse consultant's business, and there is always a chance that a competitor will be unable to complete an assignment or will not perform up to expectations, and the consultant may get a follow-up call. It is also possible that one consultant will back out of a commitment to a client, and a second consultant will get a last-minute call and engagement.

A telephone call should be given undivided attention. If the consultant cannot give the caller focused attention, schedule a telephone appointment at a mutually convenient time. Ask the caller the *who, what,* and *when* questions. The nurse consultant should take comprehensive notes for later reference.

The *who* questions should be directed toward the business or organization represented. Ask for information about the mission of the organization, the organization's goals, and key players or stakeholders. Determine the role the caller plays in the organization. This should give the nurse consultant a clue as to whether or not the caller is merely a messenger or someone who might be involved in the decision to retain the consultant.

The *what* questions follow. These should revolve around the consulting assignment. What is the nature of the assistance desired? Is the caller looking for an information expert, a planner, a facilitator, a mediator, or an advocate? Does the caller want a trainer or a problem solver? Ask the question another way: for example, "What would success look like to the caller at the end of the consultation?"

The *when* queries come next. These should focus on the time frame within which the assignment is to be completed. For example, a meeting of the board of directors or a systemwide meeting of nurse practitioners may be on the horizon as the time for a completed consultant's report. Ask the *when* questions during the early stages of the call. Many organizations call for an expert only at the last minute and want a major assignment completed in short order. Other commitments may preclude the consultant's taking on the assignment and completing it in the time desired. If so, it is important to acknowledge up front that the consultant cannot meet the desired timeline and to inquire about the flexibility of the schedule. If there is no flexibility, and the consultant is booked, the conversation may end here. Do not close the conversation without getting the prospective client's name and address. Let the potential client know that information about the consultant's services will be sent and that the consultant looks forward to being called for a future assignment. Thank the potential client for calling and express appreciation again when sending follow-up materials. The internal nurse consultant should also send a note of thanks when he or she cannot take on an assignment. The internal nurse consultant may have internal resources to refer the request to or may be able to tap someone to help with the workload to enable him or her to handle the assignment. Likewise, the external consultant may refer work to partners or colleagues.

Armed with the *who, what,* and *when,* the consultant can determine whether the assignment is within his or her area of expertise. The consultant may also have enough information to give the caller a "ball park" fee. Make sure to couch any discussion of fees as an estimate at this early stage. Discussing fees too soon may turn some clients off. The consultant may also grossly underestimate the cost of doing the job and underprice the work. Thus, the consultant will want to keep the door open to gather more information about the assignment, and to price it realistically and rationally. Some consultants suggest that a fee schedule should be discussed up front; if the consultant's fees are not in the client's ballpark, the conversation need go no further. Other consultants contend that getting to know more about the client and the project gives the consultant more of an opportunity to sell the client on the consultant and to calculate a more reasonable fee. The authors prefer taking the time to learn more about the client and the work desired, and then preparing a written proposal including a fee schedule to submit to the prospective client. If the caller insists on a price quote, consider giving a range or, perhaps, an hourly fee.

Another predicament at this early stage of inquiry is the possibility that the prospective client does not have the consulting work budgeted or the money authorized by an approving authority. The consultant can save a lot of time and work by asking a question such as, "Has this work been budgeted to be completed this year?" or "What budgetary authorization will have to be obtained to proceed with the consultation?" The answers to such questions will give the consultant a notion of whether the caller is shopping and will purchase later, if at all, or is planning to buy in the near future.

If the consultant is not qualified to handle the work or does not have the time, refer the inquirer to a competent alternative. If there is no alternative consultant to suggest, offer to locate one. Willingness to help a potential client builds goodwill and may result in the opportunity for another assignment down the road.

Referrals to colleagues are another avenue to use in building the consulting business and the consultant's networks. When referring a caller to another colleague, be sure the colleague is a competent alternative. Then follow up to find out how the consultation went. The potential client may remember the nurse consultant the next time assistance is needed. Also, be sure to call the colleague to whom the client was referred so that the colleague knows the source of the referral. In this way, a reciprocal relationship between consultants can be built.

Always thank a colleague or contact for referring business. Such a courtesy will set the nurse consultant apart. Courtesy also generates repeated referrals. For those who refer often, send business their way if it is possible and appropriate. Also, send an occasional token of appreciation.

If the assignment is one the nurse consultant has the time and talent to handle, and the caller is in the position to make a "buy" decision, begin to sell the caller. Although when making the sales pitch the consultant will have to gauge the time the potential client is willing to spend on the telephone, the following items might be included:

- Point out special expertise
- Provide information on involvement in a similar assignment (protecting the proprietary information of other clients)
- Offer a reference or two
- Convey a sense of energy and enthusiasm for the work
- Suggest several potential approaches to tackling the assignment

Consultant Interviews

On occasion, a prospective client will ask to meet the prospective consultant in person for an interview or ask the potential consultant to make a presentation. This can be a time-consuming process, and the nurse consultant will want to be sure he or she has the skills and the time to take on the assignment before agreeing to an interview or presentation. Thus, some information, such as type of project and time frame, will have to be obtained over the telephone . If an interview is agreed to, be sure to determine who will be the interviewer. Ask if this person will make the decision to engage a consultant, or if another person or group in the organization will be involved. If the answer is that others will make the decision, try to include a meeting with the others at the time the interview is scheduled.

Be clear about the date, time, and place of the interview. Ask for some basic information about the client (e.g., request a recent annual report or a copy of a recent journal or newsletter). Do homework—find out as much as possible about the organization and the people involved through material provided, library research, and the consultant's networks.

Go to the interview prepared to ask questions. Berger, Rayo and Del-Togno-Armanasco (1993, p. 67) recommend the following questions:

1. What are the objectives of the consultation (what is the client hoping to achieve)?
2. How many people will be involved in the process? How will they be selected? What is the composition of the group?
3. What is the likely time frame?
4. What facilities and assistance are available?
5. What taboos or constraints exist within the organization?

Objectives.   Ferreting out the problem, issue, or matter that needs attention is critical. Sometimes clients are not sure what the problem is, yet they know something is not working, someone is unhappy, or something is broken or will be soon. Other clients are crystal-clear about the problem or issue yet do not have a clue about how to deal with it, or, more likely, have tried to handle the matter and have not been successful. Some clients may be looking for an extra pair of hands or another good head for a period of time. Some organizations know exactly what needs to be done and want it confirmed by an expert; often, an "outside" opinion has more credibility than the opinion of those with day-to-day responsibility. Again, a good question to ask is: "What would success look like to you at the end of our work together?"

People Involved.   Tackle this question from several angles. Ask who will be involved in making the decision about the consultant. If it is a board of directors, for example, ask when the board will make the decision and if the nurse consultant might have the opportunity to meet with the board to make a brief presentation (or sales pitch). If not, any written materials or proposal the nurse consultant submits to the potential client will have to be doubly persuasive.

Also, be sure to ask if other consultants will be involved in the consultation process. One of the authors began a project with a client only to find that the client had engaged another consultant too, anticipating that both could work together to deal with the problem. If other consultants are to be involved, find out as much as possible about them. If the nurse consultant is hired for the job, be sure to talk with any other consultants engaged to work on the same activity.

Some consultants will not want to work on a project if other consultants are involved. Other consultants will view it as a challenge or just another way of doing business and will proceed accordingly. The nurse consultant will want to weigh the following considerations:

- Are the work styles and approaches of both consultants similar?
- Does the nurse consultant know the other consultant and respect his or her work?
- Is the other consultant easy to reach and communicate with?
- Will the consultation lead to other business with the client organization or with the other consultant?
- Will the client be harmed if both consultants proceed with or do not proceed with the assignment?
- Is there something to be learned—a body of knowledge or a new skill, from the other consultant?
- Will the nurse consultant be at an advantage or a disadvantage when proceeding with a joint consultation?

If the nurse consultant determines that working with another consultant is not appropriate, it will be necessary to decline the work gracefully. Care should be taken when refusing work so that the nurse consultant does not get a reputation for being unable or unwilling to work with others. If an assignment has already been accepted, it is wise to proceed with the job and make the best of it. If the consultation has not been agreed to and the nurse consultant considers it unwise to accept an engagement when another consultant is already involved, it is best to decline the work without mentioning the other consultant.

The nurse consultant should also inquire who on the organization's staff will serve as the liaison to the consultant. Ask who on the organization's staff will be involved in the consultation process; for example, who will need to be part of a training activity, or to what staff groups should training videos be geared?

Time Frame.   Although the nurse consultant may have asked about the time frame for the work at the time of the initial inquiry, ask again. Changing demands on an organization and constantly changing schedules can require a project to be put on a fast track or slowed down. Determine if there are key target dates that must be met for progress reports or for work products to be tested. If interviews are to be conducted with integral personnel, determine if these people will be available throughout the consultation period, or if they must be interviewed by or after a certain date.

Facilities and Assistance. More often than not, much of a consultant's work is done on the client's premises. The consultant will want a place to work—for example, to conduct interviews or training. Equipment such as telephone, fax, video cassette recorder, computer, or copier may be needed. Perhaps clerical or audiovisual assistance will be required. Determine initially the kinds of facilities and assistance available. Such knowledge will probably influence any proposal the consultant submits and the pricing of the consultation.

Taboos or Constraints. Knowledge of an organization's culture, pressures, and ways of doing business can save a consultant time and embarrassment. For example, the consultant who needs to schedule interviews with personnel who are preparing for a visit next week from the Joint Commission on Accreditation of Healthcare Organization (JCAHO) may save time for all by scheduling interviews following the JCAHO visit. The consultant who tries repeatedly to make a copy on the copy machine only to have bells ring and buzzers sound will be spared considerable embarrassment if he or she knows that an authorization code must be entered first. The consultant who enters a client's facility on Friday "dressed to the nines" when the entire staff is dressed for "casual day" may have a different impact from what would have happened if he or she had also observed "casual day."

Although some of these inquiries may have been made at the time of scheduling the interview, ask again. The answers may have changed. The consultant is likely to be better prepared to ask the question in more detail, and probe the answer in greater depth after doing research on the potential customer.

Go to the interview prepared to sell. The consultant is a salesperson. To make a sale, the consultant has to be a consummate listener. Listen to what the client needs and forge cordial relations with the prospective customer. At the same time, the consultant has the opportunity to build credibility primarily by listening to the client's needs and rephrasing them in the consultant's own words to be sure the consultant knows what the prospective customer has said. This translates into what the customer needs or wants. Then the consultant must match the client's needs with the product or service the consultant has to offer. The consultant must customize his or her service so that the characteristics and benefits of the service match the customer's needs.

One of the authors recalls vividly a first client interaction in which she tried to sell the client a product that clearly did not respond to the needs the client was expressing. Rather, the consultant kept trying to sell the client a package that was at odds with what the client wanted. The author has reflected on the conversation many times since and concluded that she was not listening carefully to the clues the client was giving about his needs. Rather, the consultant was trying to fit the client into a nice, tidy diagnosis for which a generic remedy could be applied. The consultant did not make a sale.

Request for Proposal

Organizations that have a complex project or body of work for which external expertise is needed will frequently issue a request for proposal (RFP). In fact, the authors have noted that even projects of a single day's duration—for example, training assignments—are increasingly coming with an RFP. A client is likely to distribute RFPs to several consultants, seeking a range of input on how an assignment might be carried out and at what fee. The RFP might arrive in the consultant's office "out of the blue" or be preceded by a call or letter of inquiry to determine if the consultant is interested in responding.

The wise consultant will read the RFP thoroughly and, if interested in responding, will make every effort to find out more about the organization seeking assistance and the details of the assignment. The organization can be called for an annual report, additional information, and responses to questions about the RFP. In addition, do as much detective work as possible. Organizations may have filed reports with various governmental agencies, such as a licensing body or secretary of state, which can be reviewed by the public. Accrediting agencies, trade or professional associations, the Better Business Bureau, and libraries are potential information sources as well. Tap into networks, both personal and professional, to determine if a colleague or contact has knowledge of or experience with the group issuing the RFP.

The *who, what,* and *when* questions are likely to be answered by a thorough review of the RFP and the accompanying letter and materials. Read the RFP and make a copy of it. Go through the RFP, completing all questions and requests for information. If the consultant has questions about the proposal, call the potential client and seek clarification. Before the call, list all questions so that the prospective client does not have to be called repeatedly. Put the completed RFP aside for a day, and then pick it up and review it to make sure responses are on target, complete, and informative. Check for punctuation and spelling errors. Remember that "spell check" on the computer is not fail-safe. Avoid acronyms and jargon. Be clear and concise, and do not oversell or undersell. The knowledge obtained about the client should help with the "sell." If the consultant has worked with the client before, the approach may be different from the one when the consultant has had no former interaction. A review of a completed RFP by a friend or colleague before submission can be a good quality check.

The RFP is also an opportunity to sell consulting services. If the consultant has tackled a similar problem or provided the same service before, say so and quantify the work and results. For example, suppose the nurse consultant worked with a long-term-care facility to reduce the incidence of falls through better room lighting, institution of a "getting up" buddy system, and use of non-skid slippers by all residents, thereby reducing falls by 64%, which, in turn, reduced the facility's liability insurance premium by $8,000. If this is applicable to the potential assignment, say so in the proposal.

The nurse consultant will probably be asked to provide references to attest to previous work. The RFP may specify the number of references required. If not, three to five references are about right. Be sure to provide references who are familiar with work that matches the specifications in the RFP. Be sure to ask those prospective references if they are willing to provide a recommendation. Also, be sure that the references are familiar with recent work and will give a good recommendation. Provide the name and title of the reference, the address, and telephone and fax numbers.

If the consultant is just starting in the business or is bidding for an assignment that matches his or her skill set but has not yet accomplished a consultation exactly like the one requested, identify those experiences that approximate the specifications. Annotate each reference, pointing out the type of consultation provided and make the linkages to the assignment under consideration—that is, make the case.

If the nurse consultant is new to the consulting business, it is likely that he or she will be asked to do things not done before. If it is possible to leverage previous experience and knowledge and handle the new assignment, do so. Do not hesitate to reach out to a trusted colleague for help or coaching, or bring in an experienced consultant to help with the assignment. (Be sure to consider this in pricing the consultation.)

If the consultation is truly beyond the consultant's experience and expertise, do not take it on. Taking business for which a consultant is not qualified and cannot competently perform sets the stage for failure as a consultant. It is also dishonest and unethical.

A short-term assignment, such as one-time training or meeting facilitation, might be agreed to over the telephone. Such an agreement should be followed up with a confirming letter restating the goals, time lines, and fees for the assignment. The confirming letter should be signed by both parties so that all are clear about what work is to be done, when the work is to be done, and how much money is involved.

A comprehensive assignment, such as an operational audit or program redesign, probably merits a detailed proposal identifying the goals of the

TABLE 2.1   Sample Statement of Project Deliverables

The deliverables for this project are:

1. Environmental scan
2. Facilitation of four focus groups of stakeholders
3. Facilitation of one focus group of staff
4. Report on the focus groups
5. Three proposed models for a statewide consortium of home care agencies
6. Business plan for the consortium, depending on the model selected
7. Implementation plan and timetable

consultation; how the assignment would be carried out; who should be available to the consultant and who, other than the consultant, will be involved in the work; the materials to which the consultant must have access; the time line, including any expected progress reports and the final report date; and the fee structure and any advance or periodic payment requirements.

A clear statement of the "deliverables" the consultant will provide should also be included in the consulting agreement (see Table 2.1). This will ensure that both the client and the consultant are clear about expectations and outcomes.

The consultant's proposal should also reflect a process to be followed in the event the assignment is terminated; for example, the payment of any outstanding expenses and the return of materials.

Negotiations

As a result of a telephone inquiry or a response to an RFP, a prospective client may want to take the next step toward engaging the consultant. It is at this stage that the terms and conditions of working together are negotiated. Negotiating is an exchange of information with an intent to resolve a problem or deal with an issue. Although negotiating is frequently thought of in terms of winners and losers, it is a process that should be used to move from "me against you" to "us against the problem."

In the survey of nurse consultants we conducted in mid-1995, negotiating contracts was one of the most common areas in which consultants needed help when they began consulting (56 of 128; 44%) and where some report they need help today (11 of 79; 14%).

Life is a series of negotiations. For example, spouses might confer and decide that one will cook dinner and the other will wash dishes. Families might debate preferred vacation sites and agree to vacation in Alaska this year and the Caribbean next year. The authors of this book conferred and agreed on the chapters each would write.

Stages in Forging an Agreement. Skopec and Kiely (1994) suggest there are four stages to forging an agreement between client and consultant:

- Relate
- Explore
- Propose
- Agree

Relate. Get to know the other party to the situation—in this case, the client. Before meeting the client, learn as much as possible from sources such as annual reports (often available on request or at the library) and consultant networks. The authors frequently ask a client for information in advance of a meeting. More often than not, the client is pleased to give a bit of history about his or her organization over the telephone and to mail or fax documents, such as informational brochures, annual reports, bylaws, or newsletters. The important point is for the consultant to set the tone for the relationship at this early stage. A consultant starts building a relationship from the first contact with the client. The first contact should be one in which the consultant establishes a climate of listening and of interest in the client and the client's problems. Such a climate will help the client feel comfortable, create a willingness to share information, and build trust and confidence in the consultant.

Explore. At this step, listening continues, and players state their positions. The client identifies the work to be done or problem to be solved, and the consultant describes products or services that might respond to the issue. Thus, the client's need is identified, and the consultant's skills are matched to the need. The client might inquire about the consultant's experience with the type of work the client needs done or the problem to be solved. The consultant may provide examples of previous work or provide references for the prospective client to contact.

The price of the consultant's services might come into play at this step. The client will want to know: "How much will it cost to solve the problem?" The consultant will want to defer the answer to this question as long as possible in an effort to gain as much information about the client's situation so as to price the product appropriately and competitively.

Propose. The consultant makes a concrete proposal to the client, restating the problem to be resolved or the matter to be tackled, the mechanism to be used in handling the problem or issue, the time line for doing the work, and the price. The proposal can be oral or in writing. The proposal should also include the consultant's skills, qualifications, and references.

Agree. This step is the meat of the matter. It is the time for creating alternatives and options, and for swapping and compromise. It is the negotiating or bargaining stage. It may result in agreement, recasting of the consultant's proposal, or no deal.

Conditions for Negotiations.   Kaine (1994) suggests that there are three conditions for negotiations:

1. The terms of a relationship can be varied. If the terms cannot be varied, the consultant is selling.
2. There is a scarce resource or what is perceived to be a scarce resource around which an understanding must be reached.
3. Each party has more to gain by negotiating than by not negotiating.

For many consultants these conditions vary greatly depending on the situation at hand. In some instances, the terms of the work under consideration—for example, the price—can be varied. In others, the consultant will not be able to vary the price of the product and will need to engage in selling.

Although consultants may not be a scarce resource per se, the skills and talents of name, or reputation of a particular consultant might be perceived as a scarce resource and, therefore, one over which a client is willing to negotiate.

Certainly, the consultant has more to gain by negotiating than not. The major gain is business. The client may also have more to gain by negotiating than not. The client's gain might be a fee concession from the consultant, more products for the fee the consultant proposed, or a shorter time line for the consultation.

The consultant must know whether getting a client to use the consultant's services requires a sales approach or a negotiation approach. Thus, information is again the key. The consultant will want to know what kind of competition exists in the marketplace that can also meet the prospective client's needs. Does the client face a buyer's market or a seller's market in terms of services needed? Does price matter to the client, or is the completion of the work in a tight time frame more important? The nurse consultant should be able to answer many of these questions as a result of the relationship-building and exploration steps of the process.

Pricing.   The biggest issue in coming to agreement with a client usually relates to fees. Fees are most often the locus of negotiations. The consultant must do homework at this stage. The consultant must know the negotiator for the client. For example, does the negotiator for the client have authority to make the final decision? If not, be prepared for a strategy often used by car salespeople—taking a price offer to a superior for an okay. This ploy usually results in a need for further negotiations because the supervisor does not agree to the proffered price. If the nurse consultant is not negotiating with the final decision maker, the consultant might expect a superior to reject the fee agreed to between the consultant and representative of the client. The consultant can be prepared for such a strategy by determining what price concessions, if any, can be made. For example, the consultant might propose eliminating three focus groups and reducing the price by $300. Also, the consultant should be sure that the original fee structure agreed to with the client's representative is a competitive price.

The consultant should ask to see any material that the client's representative will present to a final decision maker to make sure agreements are accurately reflected. The nurse consultant can offer to prepare such material and should request an opportunity to meet with the final decision maker.

Be clear about the client's needs; identify all possible work the consultant will undertake to meet the needs; know the approximate prices competitors might charge for similar work; price each step of the work the consultant will undertake to meet the needs, and then propose a package of products or services to the client. Do not highball or lowball the price, but propose a competitive price. The consultant may get a counteroffer. Some clients make a lower counteroffer, thinking there is a better deal to be had. The consultant's reaction to the counteroffer gives the client a real clue to how much the consultant is willing to give on price. If the consultant wavers, the client might surmise that the price will come down. If the nurse consultant is shocked, this reaction might relay a message to the client that the consultant is sincere about the price. If the client's counteroffer is not acceptable, offer good reasons for rejecting it. The consultant should not cut off negotiations without making his or her own counteroffer. For example, the consultant may be able to cut the price after eliminating one or two of the features of the proposal.

It is important to listen to what the client is saying. There may be a clue to the consultant's next step. If the client says a competitor's price is less, ask for the competitor's price. If the price is divulged, the nurse consultant has two choices: meet the competitor's price if it is lower, or attempt to keep negotiating. If the consultant meets the price of the competitor, a final decision must be reached by the client. If the nurse consultant tries to continue negotiations and the client is willing to do so, the nurse consultant may want to point out what sets his or her consultation services or proposal above the competition. For example, the nurse consultant might have previous experience with a similar assignment, access to special human or material resources that can be contributed to the assignment, or the ability to complete the consultation ahead of the timetable desired by the client.

Be prepared for the client who asks for "free" products or services as a concession to the consultant's price. For example, the client might ask for 10 copies of the final report, rather than the single copy the consultant proposes, or the client might ask the consultant to make an additional presentation of the final report to the hospital board of trustees. The consultant may or may not be able to provide such additional services for the quoted price. The consultant's decision will depend on time to be allocated to the project, the need for the client's business, the potential for future consulting assignments, and the value of the assignment in generating other business.

If time permits, proposed prices should be given to the client in writing and the client's counteroffers should be obtained in writing. This gives the consultant time to price the product appropriately and respond thoughtfully and carefully to counteroffers. In today's "hurry up and do it" world, however, price negotiations are most likely to take place over the telephone.

As an aside, the authors have noted a decreasing tendency for clients to want to negotiate price. The authors think the competitiveness of the consulting field makes it a buyer's market and that potential clients are doing a lot of comparison shopping at the outset.

Steps in Negotiation. Shea (1983) suggests that negotiation might follow the steps commonly used for problem solving:

1. Define the problem or clarify the issue
2. Determine the facts
3. Identify possible solutions
4. Evaluate the options identified
5. Select the option or options best suited to the problem
6. Implement the option or options
7. Evaluate and make adjustments as necessary

Define the problem.   Parties to a negotiation bring to the table their own views about the issue to be confronted or problem to be resolved. The problem is defined by each party's perceptions and experiences. When the parties to a negotiation do not take the time to flesh out a problem or to seek mutual understanding about how the problem is defined, each participant believes firmly that his or her own perception is the right one and positions begin to harden around one-sided views. As Shea (1988) notes, each party then begins to focus on giving up as little as possible.

Clarity about the problem under consideration and a mutual understanding or definition of the problem can lead parties from a mind-set of "me against you" to "us against the problem." Focusing on the problem rather than the parties to the problem should be the goal in any negotiation.

For the nurse consultant and the prospective client, the problems are the following:

- What is the consultation required or desired?
- What are the limitations or parameters for the consultation?
- What are the fees involved?

Identify the facts. Putting together all the facts surrounding a problem can be tough work. It is easy to get lost in extraneous matters, or to conjure up old hurts or wrongs. A dispassionate approach to identifying the relevant concerns of each party is essential. Facts should not be confused with assumptions, nor should inferences be drawn from the facts. Shea (1988) suggests that each party collect the significant facts and hold them until the stage of the process where options for solutions to the problem are evaluated. At the first step, the nurse consultant will want to learn as much as possible about the client and the client's needs.

Identify possible solutions. At this stage, the parties should identify as many potential solutions to the problem as possible. All ideas should be welcome and, at this stage, none should be judged good or bad, or right or wrong. The idea is to get as many creative notions about resolving the problem onto the table. At this stage, the nurse consultant identifies possible approaches, strategies, and options for the consultation. Approaches and options may be priced as an aggregate package or separately priced.

Evaluate the solutions identified. This step is one in which the possible solutions to the problem can be identified. At this stage, the possible solutions should be weighed and measured against the mutually defined problem and the facts. Although feelings may surface in this step, it is a stage in which logic, common sense, and good judgment should prevail. The first three steps should have moved the parties to an "us against the problem" view of the situation. Step three is also a step during which client and consultant work through the approaches to the consultation and the price.

Select the solution. The solution or combination of solutions for the problem should be selected at this stage. The conclusion should be one that all parties can accept and commit themselves to implementing. At this step, the consultant is either hired or dropped.

Implement the solution. How the solution will be carried out is almost as important as the solution itself. Failure to decide how to implement the solution can cause confusion and can make best-intentioned parties back away from a mutual agreement on what to do to solve a problem. The *how* should be discussed and agreed to in much the way as the *what* was selected—that is, brainstorm implementation options, weigh and measure them against the solution and any relevant facts, and select the implementation approach that best fits the situation. If the consultant is hired, the consultation ensues.

Evaluate. The parties to a negotiation will want to determine how the solution and its implementation are going. Milestones or benchmarks may help parties answer the question of, "How are we doing?" At this stage, it is most likely that the nurse consultant will evaluate his or her acumen in negotiating or securing a client.

The nurse consultant will want to ask the following:

1. How did I do?
2. What did I learn?
3. What will I do differently in the future?

As noted earlier, negotiation is often perceived as a process with winners and losers. Given this mind-set, the consultant's goal would be for him or her to win and for the client to lose. Conversely, the client's goal would be to win, which means that the consultant loses. The reader will properly conclude that no consultant will stay in business long if the consultant wants to win at the expense of a client. The client is not going to trust or hire any consultant who wants the client to lose.

Rules for Negotiating. Kaine (1994, pp. 64–71) reports eight rules for dealing with a conflict during negotiations:

1. Avoid escalating a conflict.
2. Know when to walk away.
3. Be a careful communicator.
4. Realize that no one wins an argument.
5. Lead by questioning.
6. Avoid making counterproposals.
7. Focus on your strongest points.
8. Settle on an agreement that is workable.

Avoid escalating a conflict. Kaine (1994) notes that the person who speaks first sets the tone for the negotiation. A positive tone can lead to building trust, sharing information, and establishing a real interest in solving the problem. Thus, the nurse consultant should take the opportunity to identify the conflict dispassionately when it arises and ascertain whether or not the client has the same understanding of the conflict. The nurse consultant might also provide information that can minimize or resolve the conflict. The nurse consultant should maintain an even temper and make a genuine appeal for resolution of the problem.

Walk away. If the consultant encounters angry or negative behavior or bullies, he or she should walk away. Kaine (1994) suggests that skilled negotiators can make conflict work in their favor by demonstrating that they cannot be pushed around. In fact, Kaine (1994) recommends walking away from negative or angry behavior as a way to deal with people bent on pushing others around. Walking away will be difficult for the consultant to do, as it may mean a lost opportunity. But if an individual cannot leave a conflict, he or she loses power (Kaine, 1994).

Be a careful communicator. Skilled negotiators announce what they are going to say, say it, and then announce what they have said. Kaine (1994) suggests that labeling communication lends clarity to the negotiating process and creates receptivity. For example, the nurse consultant might say, "I'd like to restate the problem you've just outlined to be sure I understand it." The nurse consultant then restates the problem. In this statement, the consultant has described what is being done in an effort to achieve clarity and receptivity.

No one wins an argument. Arguments are usually surrounded by negative terminology, such as "you're wrong" and "I disagree." Such statements drive negotiators farther away from problem resolution. Kaine (1994) reports that the skilled negotiator asks questions about the point of disagreement. For example, the nurse consultant might ask questions that begin with *how, where,* or *what.*

One of the authors recently worked with a client who wanted a key set of assumptions removed from a report. Rather than argue over whether or not the assumptions should remain in the report, the author asked the client several questions. "How will the readers of the report know on what the consultant's recommendations were based?" After several similar questions, it became obvious that the real problem was not the assumptions per se but how they were stated. The author, not unlike a skilled negotiator, proposed a restatement of the assumptions that was accepted with minor changes. As Kaine (1994) points out "skilled negotiators realize they must first educate, then negotiate" (p. 65).

Lead by questioning. Ever notice how those famous detectives like Jessica Fletcher or Inspector Clouseau ask many questions long before reaching conclusions? Why? Questions lead to information, including potential clues to solve a mystery or a murder. The consummate negotiator will also ask questions to gain understanding, information, and clues. Questions are a way to restate issues, to clarify, and to test comprehension. Questions are also a great way to reflect back what someone else has just said. Hearing information repeated through a question can cause people to drop a matter or change their minds. Questions also give the negotiator time to think through what has just been said, and to contrast and compare it with already known information.

The nurse consultant will avoid asking questions that can be answered "yes" or "no." Such questions usually begin with the word "do." For example, "Do you have a problem with the fee proposed?" The answer will most certainly be yes or no. If the answer is yes, the consultant will not get any additional information or clues about the problem. Ask instead, "What are the problems with the proposal?" or "How does the fee coincide with what you had planned to pay for this work?" Valuable information is likely to be revealed that gives the nurse consultant ideas for responding to any shortcomings in the proposal or the fee structure.

Avoid making counterproposals.   Kaine (1994) suggests that responding to a proposal with a counterproposal is not a good bargaining strategy. Rather, he urges the negotiator to ask questions about the proposal to elicit its shortcomings and then suggest ways to resolve the shortcomings. Thus, the negotiator has advanced solutions to problems identified rather than making counterproposals that miss the mark and set the stage for a consultant-versus-client situation rather than consultant and client against the problem.

Focus on your strongest positions.   Strong points or reasons should be the focal point of discussions. Flimsy or fragile arguments tend to draw the focus away from the strong positions to weaker matters that can be diversionary.

Settle on a workable agreement.   Be sure all parties to the negotiation understand what has been agreed to and how the agreement will be carried out. This is the time to ask what problems might occur in implementing the agreement and then agree on how such problems will be handled. For example, the consultant might ask the client, "What are the likely roadblocks we will run into during the consultation?"

Contracts

An agreement or contract sets forth the work to be done by the consultant and the amount the consultant will be paid for the work. Cohen (1991) suggests that the elements of any contract are the *who, what, where, when,* and *how much.*

Who. This section of the contract, usually section 1, identifies the parties to the contract. The name of the nurse consultant or the nurse consultant's firm and the name of the client are included in this portion of the contract. Any other individuals or companies involved in the consultation should also be identified in this section. The roles of the other parties should be outlined, as well as to whom the parties are accountable. For example, the section might state that the High Numbers Research Firm will gather and analyze all statistical data and will report and be accountable to the Top-Notch Consulting Firm.

What. The next section identifies the products or services the nurse consultant will provide the client.

Where. This section identifies the place where the consultation services are to be provided. If the services are to be provided on the client's premises, the address of the premises should be included. If the nurse consultant will provide services at satellite clinics, the identity of the clinics and the addresses of the clinics should be included.

When. A timetable for the steps of the consultation should be included in this section. If dates are established for interim reports, the dates should be included in this section. The date for the final product to be provided to the client should be noted in this portion of the agreement. The fee payment schedule should also be included in this section.

Some agreements include a provision in the contract for termination of the services by either the client or the consultant. Such a stipulation is a safeguard for client and consultant in that the parameters of dissolving a consulting relation are established at the outset of the work. Language should cover payment to the consultant for work done or expenses incurred up to the date of termination of the contract. Language might also be included to require the consultant to return all proprietary information to the client.

How Much. The fee the consultant will receive for the services provided should be included in this section. If the consultant is to be reimbursed for out-of-pocket expenses, such as parking, postage, or mileage, reimbursement for such direct expenses should be noted in this section.

PLANNING

A written agreement for the consultation is now in place including the "drop dead" date for completion of the work. Sit down with the client and review the goals of the consultation, time lines, information needed, access to key people, fees, and payment schedules—and the parameters for termination of work, if necessary.

Planning for each step of the consulting assignment now begins. Pull out the proposal submitted to get the job, and the agreed-on contract. No doubt, these documents provide a time line for certain elements of the project. In fact, some consultants include as an integral part of their proposals a flowchart or timetable that outlines each step of the project. Such a chart or timetable can be most helpful at the planning stage. Taking the date for completion of the assignment, some consultants prefer to plan backward, outlining each step of the process required to get to the end result: assigning a time frame for the work and a date for completion of each step. It is important to review, flesh out, and revise each step during the planning phase.

Occasionally, what the client really wants and what the consultant thought he or she was hired to do differ. Confirm the purpose of the consultation through discussion of goals and expectations. Be specific, and use "I" questions. This puts the onus for understanding the assignment on the nurse consultant and neutralizes the sense of threat that can potentially arise when the nurse consultant uses the word "you." From time to time, employees or staffs of organizations will resist "outside" help. Thus, it is important to assume a persona that is nonthreatening, friendly, and focused from the outset.

Be sure to determine who in the organization will be the consultant's primary contact. A primary contact can help the consultant weave through processes, procedures, systems, and roadblocks with dispatch. A key liaison can provide access to information, staff, and others pivotal to helping the nurse consultant with the assignment. The liaison can respond to questions and guide the consultant through the organizational processes and structures.

Tie down time frames for deliverables. Be clear about what is expected and when. If the nurse consultant is going to have trouble with prescheduled meeting dates because of other work, say so and be prepared with alternatives. For example, the consultant might meet with a key committee the evening before a prescheduled meeting or participate in a portion of the meeting by conference call in lieu of attending the entire meeting.

Completing an assignment on time may require the use of an associate. If the consultant involves others in the consulting assignment, let the client know who will be working with the consultant, how and when the helper will be involved, and what the qualifications of the aide are. It is wise to stipulate in the agreement with the client that the consultant can bring in others to help with the assignment. In some instances, the nurse consultant may want to give the client permission to review and comment on any associates brought to the job. It is also important that any fee agreed to include all the human resources needed for the consulting assignment. No one wants a surprise like an additional cost once the consultation is under way. It is up to the nurse consultant to anticipate the talent needed before agreeing to fees or to the time line for the work to be done.

Another caution is to be sure that the principal taking the assignment remains the principal on the consulting job. Too many clients have been alienated and too much credibility has been lost by consultants who take a job and then turn it over to a junior partner. A client often consciously buys the reputation and "name" of a consultant as well as the expert's competence, skills, and expertise.

Identify and gather all the information about the client needed to do the job. Information might include strategic plans, budgets, articles of incorporation, bylaws, organizational charts, newsletters, journals, accreditation or licensing reports, marketing plans and materials, risk management reports, position statements, policies, and job descriptions. It is wise to stipulate in a consulting agreement the kinds of information to which the consultant will have access. Query the client to identify information that might be helpful in doing the job. Information should be kept confidential and may need to be returned to the client on completion of the work.

The consultant must do his or her homework. Review all relevant materials, prepare questions, and identify issues to be raised while on the client's premises. Identify and schedule appointments with key individuals integral to helping with the consulting work. The organization's staff will be critical to helping with the consulting assignment, but people external to the organization should not be overlooked. Board members, customers, vendors, and suppliers may be integral to the consulting task. Identification of and access to individuals is another aspect of a consulting assignment that should be crystallized, clarified, and agreed to before the assignment begins. Be on the lookout for those who might hold different viewpoints. Do not settle for those who will give the "party line." Speaking with those who are not a part of the client's immediate "family" (i.e., employees, board members, committee members, legal counsel, and accountants) should generally be cleared with the client first. Clients may not want others to know the consultation is under way, for any number of reasons (e.g., protection of trade secrets, competitive advantage, preservation of reputation or safekeeping of proprietary information).

When interviewing individuals related to the consulting duty, the nurse consultant should identify himself or herself and the reason for requesting an interview. Be clear about the goals of the consultation and assure the interviewee that information received will be kept confidential. If information is divulged that should be quoted in a report or followed up, ask the person's permission to print a quote, repeat a fact, or follow up with other sources for clarity. Much information can be aggregated, making the identity of the source unnecessary. On the other hand, a workable idea for problem resolution or a new venture should be attributed to the source. Consultants who use others' work, including ideas, without giving credit are stealing; they are practicing unethically and are headed for trouble, not to mention a guilty conscience.

From time to time, an employee or individual associated with a client will attempt to establish a more personal relationship with the consultant. This might take the form of asking for a special meeting to discuss an aspect of the assignment that is not relevant to the person asking. Inappropriate interactions might also take the form of an attempt to influence the data gathered or the outcomes reported. All objectivity and credibility is on the line when a consultant becomes inappropriately involved with a client's employee or other representatives. A consultant's reputation is at stake with every client contact, so it is best to remain businesslike and focused on the assignment.

IMPLEMENTATION OR INTERVENTION

Now the work begins in earnest. In this stage, the consultant has secured the job, is clear about the problem to be tackled or the service to be provided, has a plan in place, and is ready to go to work.

Step 1: Review

Review the goals of the consultation and the products to be achieved or the services to be provided. Take the work plan that has been refined, and review the agreed-on deliverables and time lines in the contract again. Although this review may seem duplicative, it is important in that the nurse consultant will probably have several projects under way at once, and periodic review of the goals and outcomes will help keep the consultant focused and on schedule.

Step 2: "Desk Audit"

A well-known consulting firm refers to this step as the "desk audit." Give careful attention to learning as much about the client as possible. In the planning phase, the consultant requested several materials for review pertinent to the assignment. An organizational liaison was identified. The consultant should review all materials provided and notes from any meetings or interviews that took place leading to or negotiating the contract. A list of questions or inquiries in areas of uncertainty, including a list of additional references or documents needed, should be prepared.

Step 3: Clarification and Introductions

Meet with the client liaison by telephone or in person to clarify questions; request additional materials; and gather the names, telephone and fax numbers, and addresses of those to be interviewed or visited during the consultation. At this step, the consultant may collaborate with the client to prepare a letter of introduction to those in the client's "family" who will be interviewed or who might be visited as a part of the fieldwork or are an integral part of developing a training activity. Such a letter introduces the consultant and identifies the goals of the consultation and the reasons for interviews or visits. Others outside the "family" who are to be included as a part of the data-gathering process should receive a telephone call or a letter of introduction from the client and consultant as well.

Step 4: Research and Data Collection

At this stage, interviews are conducted, field visits are made, research is carried out, or data are gathered. Perhaps library research is done, brainstorming sessions are held, and ideas are generated. At this step, the timetable should be reviewed again to make sure the consultation is proceeding as planned. A report on work in progress may be given to the client. By the way, due dates for progress reports may be a part of the contract with the client.

If the timetable needs to be revised, it is at this stage that it becomes obvious. For example, people to be interviewed are sometimes not available at the time agreed to or cannot be contacted. Telephone tag can be a real impediment at this stage of work. A field visit may have to be rescheduled because of an emergency in a facility to be visited. Any foreseen difficulty in meeting an agreed on timeline for work to be done should be identified and examined, and the consultant should determine what might be done to correct the difficulty. For example, consider the following:

- Can another individual who is easier to contact be substituted for an interview?
- Can a different facility be visited?
- Can the consultant proceed to other areas of the assignment and return later to the area where there is delay?

In other words, the consultant should make every possible effort to control the situation and adhere to the timetable. It may be appropriate to let the client know of the difficulties, including suggestions as to how they might be handled.

A word about interviews is in order here. Both the external and the internal consultant will find matters of confidentiality important to deal with, because people's views, issues, problems, complaints, or ideas are often well known throughout an institution. An assurance of anonymity to those to be interviewed often opens doors to information that the consultant might find helpful. Such an assurance should be given at the time the consultant is introduced to those to be interviewed. Those who have engaged the consultant must concur at the beginning of the process that the consultant will not be asked to divulge confidences. In some instances, those interviewed about the use of a product, application of a technique, or data—or those with a "gem" of an idea—will want recognition. Still, permission to recognize or make attribution of an idea or opinion should be obtained by the consultant before divulging a particular viewpoint.

Step 5: Preliminary Findings

Preliminary findings or ideas begin to crystallize. Identification of additional data needed or research to be done should also occur at this step and such work should be carried out. Again, the timetable should be reviewed, and any foreseen problems handled.

Step 6: Analysis

Results are analyzed. Preliminary recommendations are developed and may be tested or tried out against any predetermined criteria set for the consultation. Field or pilot tests of a new or revised process or procedure or product might occur.

Preliminary findings and recommendations might be appropriate to share or test with the client to ensure that the work is on target. In the authors' experience, sharing preliminary findings and recommendations with a client pays dividends. Errors can be caught and corrected, missing links found and connected, "hot spots" identified, data amplified, and misunderstandings rectified.

Sharing preliminary findings with clients can be a disadvantage, however, as when a client asks that findings or recommendations be changed or removed. This may be an ethical dilemma for the consultant. First, the consultant should be clear about the client's request. It may be that there is a bothersome word that can be changed, or one of the findings may no longer be true, or one of the recommendations may already be implemented. The consultant must ask if the client's request distorts the recommendations or compromises the consultant's work. If the answer is a clear yes, the consultant will probably not make the change requested. If the answer is no or maybe, the consultant may want to make the change or work further with the client on the issue.

As an example, one of the authors completed a compensation consultation and presented the findings and recommendations to a client. The client was taken aback to learn that the organization's staff had perceived a one-time benefit as a permanent benefit and that the consultant had considered the benefit in calculating the aggregate compensation package. The matter was clarified at all levels of the organization, and the consultant restated the findings and recommendations.

Step 7: Report

This step is usually the one in which a final report or product is prepared for the client and presented.

Format of Report.   The report format will, in part, be dictated by the work being done. For example, if the consultation outcome is a training program for volunteer caregivers to provide respite services for families of people in hospices, the report is likely to be a training curriculum and, perhaps, the actual conduct of the training. If the consulting assignment was to prepare a grant proposal to submit to a foundation to build and equip a children's hospital, the report will be the completed grant proposal.

The consultant should advise the client of the format the consultant will use for any written report. If the client has a preferred format or special requirements for a report, the consultant can consider these.

Although there are several formats that can be used in crafting a final report, one international association consulting firm observes the following format; to this we would add a table of contents.

1. Overview
2. Methodology
3. Observations and findings
4. Recommendations
5. Implementation plan and timetable
6. Summary
7. Addenda

Overview.   The overview is an introduction that includes the purpose and focus of the project. It might provide a bit of information about the client—for example, the client's relevant history, the mission of the client organization, the environment within which the client operates, and recognition of any key personnel in the client organization who have been integral to the conduct of the consultation. The client's liaison might be thanked for special assistance provided or insights offered.

Methodology.   The approach used in carrying out the consulting assignment is described in this section. If a study was conducted, the methodology might include information about document review or a literature search, interviews conducted or focus groups held, surveys distributed, tests performed, and so forth. Quantifying numbers should be cited. For example, 110 nursing assistants participated in focus groups, 60 registered nurses were interviewed individually, 50 surveys were distributed to physicians, and 30 surveys were returned. To take another example, 70 school nurses in 10 school systems tested the apnea monitors.

The methodology section sets the stage for the findings and recommendations. It must be constructed in such a way as to be credible and clear. It may need to be backed up with addenda (see below) that include items such as survey instruments, focus-group questions, more detailed test data, statistical analysis, or amplification of field research.

Observations and findings.   Observations and findings include research results, measurements, perceptions, what was noticed or what was not noticed, what was heard or went unsaid, and results of inspections or tests. Qualitative and quantitative approaches might be taken in presenting this section. Visual displays, such as charts or graphs, might be used to depict discoveries.

Recommendations.   The recommendations section of the report contains the suggestions of the consultant about how to handle the observations and findings. In other words, the consultant answers the question, "What should be done about what was found?"

Implementation plan and timetable.   Not every consultant's report will include this kind of guidance, the client may decide whether or not this advice is wanted. However, a section can go a long way toward helping the client see and understand how the recommendations might be dealt with and in what time frame. An implementation plan and a timetable are one way for the consultant to support the client in dealing with the outcomes of the consultation. A plan and timetable might provide the impetus the client needs in dealing with the recommendations.

Thus clients should be urged to take the plan and timetable, and they should also make it their own. A plan and timetable can be customized during the draft stage of report writing or soon after the client receives the consultant's report. Consultants may want to offer this service as a distinct part of the consultation package and price the package accordingly. Note, though, that the provision of an implementation plan and timetable is a value-added service and might be given up if price concessions are required.

Summary, addenda, contents. A final report should also include a contents page for ease in using the report and an executive summary that can be used by the casual reader, for a broader distribution than the complete report, or for use in a newsletter or other publication. A final report often contains addenda that provide information or background on the consultant or consulting firm; sample survey instruments or focus-group questions; tabulated results of a study; data analysis; and other information that enhances, clarifies, or justifies the recommendations in the report.

The final report must be written in such a way as to be clear and understandable. Most of the American public still reads at an eighth-grade level. Thus, it is incumbent on the consultant to know the audience for which the report is being written. Writing for a group of chemists or engineers is different from writing for a group of attorneys or nursing assistants. Every profession or occupation has a language of its own, so be careful when using acronyms and jargon. Define acronyms; it is particularly important to spell out those acronyms that are outside the field in which the consultation is occurring. For example, when writing a report for teachers or travel agents, do not suggest that the recommendations be implemented "stat." Instead, suggest that the recommendations be implemented "immediately."

Strategies for writing a report are similar to those used for preparing an oral presentation. Holtz recommends keeping the following in mind: "It's not the writer's responsibility to understand what you write; it is your responsibility to see to it that you can be easily understood" (1993, p. 302).

Reports cannot be developed overnight. Careful attention to shaping the report is a must. The authors find it helpful to prepare an outline before writing a report. Iterations of the outline are subsequently prepared and filled in with key thoughts, notes, findings, and ideas, and the report begins to take shape. A first draft of the report is written and set aside for at least 24 hours. The draft is read and improved, set aside, and read and improved again until the author is satisfied that the report is ready to be read by someone else. Cold reading of a report by a colleague or another expert in the field is a good strategy to use to be certain the report is easily understood. (The authors used such a practice in writing this book, thus unearthing valuable insights and suggestions from each other.)

Care must be taken not to share a client's confidences or information inappropriately when using another reader. In some instances, the client liaison might serve as an initial reader, providing a critique on the readability of the document rather than its contents. An associate or assistant used by the consultant during the assignment can also be tapped to review the report. If the consultant does not have the use of an independent reader and will have to rely on personal judgment as to the clarity and readability of the report, it is critical to write the report and then set it aside for a time to be reviewed later with fresh eyes.

Presenting the Report.   At this final step of the intervention-implementation process, presentation of the final report is often required. In many respects, the consultant is selling the report, particularly the recommendations. The tips in this section are also applicable to a presentation that might be called for at the beginning of the process, when the consultant is required to make a presentation to sell consulting services to get the assignment.

Block (1981) suggests the following steps in presenting a report or the results of a consultation:

1. Review purpose of the consultation or assignment.
2. Outline the agenda for the presentation meeting.
3. Present the recommendations.
4. Ask for client's reaction to findings.
5. Ask for client's reaction to recommendations.
6. Halfway through the meeting, check with the client to be sure the client is getting what is wanted.
7. Decide to proceed or stop.
8. Test for client's control and commitment.
9. Ask yourself if you got all that you wanted.
10. Give support to the client.

Purpose of the consultation.   Review the reason for the project, consultation, assignment, or work done. State what the client wanted and what the nurse consultant agreed to do. Do not give a lengthy diatribe on how the consultant and the client got together. Save time for the meat of the report and the client's response. For example, the consultant might state: "The Do Right Consulting Firm was asked to investigate the retraining needs of staff nurses to assist them in moving from the hospital practice setting to a community practice setting. Do Right did not examine related issues, such as decreased hospital occupancy rates, hospital mergers, acquisitions, or closures."

Meeting agenda. Describe how the meeting will proceed and the time sequence for the meeting. This strategy helps the consultant control the flow of the meeting. The agenda gives the audience a preview of what is to come, and a signal that reactions will be sought and that the consultant is concerned about meeting the client's needs.

Present the diagnosis and recommendations. Give the findings and suggestions for dealing with the findings. Some consultants combine these two steps; others are more circumscribed, presenting all of the data and then all of the findings. The authors are increasingly using the strategy of presenting a finding or cluster of findings and then what to do about them. Audiences seem to have a clearer understanding of the work when the diagnosis is followed by a prescribed treatment regimen. Such an approach has a risk in that a controversial diagnosis or treatment might deter attention from the aggregate data and recommendations. Control of the meeting by the consultant, including ample opportunity for client's reactions, should minimize this risk.

Client's reactions. Purposefully asking for the client's reactions to the data and then to the recommendations keeps the consultant in charge of the meeting. Reactions to the diagnosis and the treatment might occur in two steps or combined into one. The audience and the nature of the report are likely to dictate how the consultant handles this portion of the meeting.

Block (1981) suggests that getting the client's reaction is the heart of the meeting. Reactions signal the client's commitment to following up on the consultant's recommendations once the consultant leaves. Reactions are a good way to elicit resistance on the part of the group, even a small part of the group, that are then known to all and can be dealt with and perhaps overcome. Block (1981) also notes this is a time when the client's reactions might elicit a defensive tendency in the consultant, and a temptation to back away from findings and recommendations. Do not fall into this trap. The nurse consultant was retained on the basis of his or her expertise and should adhere to the recommendations provided. This stage of the meeting can be a particularly challenging time for the internal consultant, who may see members of the audience day after day or whose supervisor might be in the audience. It can also be difficult if the consultant is recommending a "new order" of things when those who created and supported the "old order" are in the room.

Is the client getting what is wanted? Few consultants take this step. Block (1981) suggests that it is one of the most significant things a consultant can do. If the client is disappointed, the consultant has time to recover or recapture the client's interest and attention, which is easier to do in the middle of the meeting than at the end. As Block (1981) notes, the client and consultant are often so caught up in the diagnosis and treatment that they fail to take the time to ask each other how the meeting is going and if the client is getting what is wanted. This can also be another defensive time for the consultant. In the author's experience, if the meeting is not going well, this most likely has to do with resistance to the recommendations, terror at having to make changes, fear of failure, or denial of problems. The consultant must also guard against the temptation to "throw in the towel."

Proceed or stop?   If the client is not getting what is wanted, the consultant has to decide whether or not to proceed with the meeting. Perhaps the best way to deal with this decision is to confront the matter head-on with the client and decide together how to proceed. For example, one of the authors recently asked a client if the organization was getting what it wanted from the meeting. The response was, "Oh yes, we got more than we asked for—from the meeting and from the report." Although there was agreement to proceed with the meeting, the consultant was signaled that the client was concerned about the data and was likely to be a real problem with implementing any of the recommendations. The consultant, thinking the findings and recommendations were right on target, was disappointed in the group's reaction and struggled to keep focused on the report and recommendations and to maintain a level of enthusiasm for the change and support for the client.

Client's control and commitment.   At this step, the consultant inquires about the client's reaction to the treatment recommended. Block (1981, p. 184) suggests a direct question such as, "Is the solution we discussed something that really makes sense to you?" To return to the example noted earlier, the author asked the audience if the solutions proposed made sense and if the client would go ahead with the treatment prescribed or if the client was uneasy about doing so. The client's commitment was low. Although there was discussion about the client's uneasiness, the client was unable to manage the uneasiness and decided to exercise control by delaying a decision on the recommendations until later. In fact, the client referred the consultant's report to a task force, and, as of the writing of this book, the task force cannot agree on the disposition of the recommendations.

Did the consultant get what was wanted?   Although this may seem like a strange question, it is at this stage of the consultation that the evaluation component of the process begins. It is a good time to ask for feedback on what the consultant might have done to be more effective. For example, the consultant might ask, "What might I have done differently to enhance your understanding of the findings and recommendations?" or "What information might I have provided that would have helped you manage your uneasiness about the recommendations?"

This is also a good time to suggest further involvement with the client, such as a contract to implement the findings or to provide the training called for in the recommendations. Broaching the subject of continued involvement with the client is a delicate matter. Some consultants use the strategy of trying to make the client so dependent on the consultant that further work is assured. Actually, the consultant, like a nurse working with a patient, should seek to make the client as self-sufficient as possible. On the other hand, the consultant should be as supportive to the client as possible in making changes prescribed. Thus, the consultant will have to weigh and measure if recommending future work together is appropriate. One well-known association consulting firm offers a 6-month checkup to clients, knowing that the momentum to make changes or implement recommendations often needs a boost or further clarification. Although this checkup is offered as an option for a small additional fee at the time the initial contract is signed, it is often only at the time the findings and recommendations are presented that the client realizes more help is needed. The consultant may then be asked about a follow-up assignment.

Such an assignment should be described clearly in a letter of agreement or contract and priced accordingly. Often the client will want a price break, believing a follow-up assignment can be done more quickly and easily by the consultant who is already knowledgeable about the organization and familiar with the recommended course of action. The consultant should evaluate the pricing structure of the follow-up assignment on the basis of amount of work involved and outcomes or products expected. A price break may be warranted in the interest of good will and marketing even if it is not warranted in terms of the work to be undertaken.

Give support. Implementing the recommendations from a consultation is the most difficult part of the process for the client. The consultant who recognizes this difficulty and who provides support for the implementation process at the time of presenting the report to the client puts a more realistic face on the consultation process and on the job to be done. As noted earlier, an implementation plan and a timetable are one way to support the client, as is the offer of a 6-month checkup. Often the authors will call a client at intervals after the consultation to check on progress.

One of the drawbacks to consulting is working with a client, completing a project, and then not knowing what happened with what was recommended. A follow-up call can relieve the desire to know, but be prepared for bad news as well as good news. Follow-up calls or inquiries are also an important marketing tool for the consultant.

EVALUATION

In the daily practice of nursing, the nurse is often present to evaluate or be part of the actual change process of making a change. For example, the nurse might observe a client's adherence to a treatment protocol, assess whether or not the client understands goals for change, and detect flagging commitment in working toward change. In consulting, the external consultant is often not present to monitor changes to be made or get feedback on implementing the consultant's recommendations. The internal consultant may or may not be a part of the implementation or follow-up process.

Process Evaluation

The connection formed between client and consultant at the outset of the relationship will influence not only their working together but any weighing of results or outcomes. If a mutuality in the relationship has developed—a give-and-take, a respect for each other's opinion and knowledge, an attention to "how we're doing" throughout the consulting process—then evaluation really has been ongoing throughout the consultation. Such evaluation is often referred to in the nursing lexicon as *process* or *formative evaluation*.

Summative Evaluation

A *summative evaluation*, by contrast, is a measuring of the outcomes or end product. Although this is not customary, the consultant and client would do well to meet at the end of the consultation for the definitive purpose of evaluating their work together. In addition, the client and consultant should each evaluate the consultation independently. The process should not be a protracted one; and it should be a process of growth, not of looking for who or what to blame. Perlov (1993) suggests that the following four questions get to the crux of the matter in summative evaluation:

1. How did we do?
2. What did we learn?
3. How did we grow?
4. How did we help others grow?

How Did We Do?   Client and consultant should tackle this question, trying to see how well the goals of the consultation were achieved. Were communications clear between both parties? Were time lines met on both sides? Did both commit adequate resources to the undertaking?

The answers to these questions may reveal flaws, errors, or missteps. Such discoveries should lead consultant and client to ask, "What are we going to do about it?"

What Did We Learn?   The data–gathering and observation phase of the consultation might be highlighted. Any insights gleaned by either client or consultant about the process or outcomes should be shared.

How Did We Grow?   This question is perhaps the most painful, as it deals with change. Perhaps the question should be, "What did we change?" or "How did we change?" The client and consultant should search for changes in behavior that were made; learning that occurred; risks that were taken (perhaps the consultation itself); old habits that were cast off; and openness to opinions and insights or to findings and observations.

How Did We Help Others Grow?   Leaders in organizations who are often the consultant's client may or may not recognize and implement their responsibility for the growth of others—employees, colleagues, boards, and volunteers. A consultation is the perfect time to include key stakeholders in the process, which in itself will probably produce growth. In conducting strategic planning activities with organizations, the authors have frequently heard, "Gosh, I've never thought about the future in that way before" or "I've never done this before, but I'd like to learn. Would you help me?"

Likewise, the consultant does not always view the consultation as an opportunity to contribute to the growth of others. Consciously asking the question should heighten awareness in this area and, perhaps, willingness to do something about it. One of the key questions the consultant should ask is, "What did I contribute to the client's ability to implement the recommendations I made?" or, more bluntly, "Have I enabled the client to move ahead independently of me?"

The authors acknowledge that evaluation is potentially a risky matter for the consultant. It may mean redoing some work; acknowledging frailty; or, more likely, a change in behavior for the next time. Evaluation is, however, an undertaking the consultant should assume even if it does not include the client. Evaluation can enhance the consultant's awareness of performance, heighten resolve to make changes if necessary, and often show the way to make those changes.

SUMMARY

The consultation process, like the nursing process, is one of problem solving. The act of consultation is one that nurses use every day when caring for patients, collaborating with colleagues or clients, and forging community relationships or personal partnerships. The nurse consultant and the client are both winners when an orderly assessment and diagnosis of a problem or situation occurs, collaborative planning for the consulting assignment ensues, appropriate and adequate intervention or implementation takes place, and evaluation follows.

REFERENCES

Berger, M. C., Ray, L. N., & Del Togno-Armanasco, V. (1993). The effective use of consultants. *Journal of Nursing Administration, 23,* 67.

Block, P. (1981). *Flawless consulting.* San Diego: Pfeiffer & Co.

Cohen, W. (1991). *How to make it big as a consultant* (2nd ed.). New York: AMACOM.

Holtz, H. (1993). *How to succeed as an independent consultant* (3rd ed.). New York: John Wiley & Sons.

Kaine, J. (1994). How to be negotiator-in chief. *Association Management, 46* (Suppl.: *Leadership*), L-63–71.

Perlov, D. (1993). Personal papers. New York.

Shea, G. (1988). *Creative negotiating.* Boston: CBI.

Skopec, E., & Kiely, L. (1994). *Everything's negotiable . . . when you know how to play the game.* New York: AMACOM.

3

Preparation for Consultation: Planning a Career Path

Most nurses who become consultants do not initially plan to do so. Many, like the authors, find themselves in job situations that no longer are satisfying and decide to go out on their own. Many of the 128 respondents (49, or 38%) in the survey of nurse consultants conducted by the authors in mid-1995 stated that they started consulting on their own initiative. Interestingly, another 23 (18%) were encouraged to start consulting by a colleague; fewer (20, or 16%) were encouraged by another consultant.

Only a few individuals deliberately choose to start a consulting business, setting strategy into place long before they become nurse entrepreneurs. However, most nurses do decide that they want something else besides the position they currently hold in a hospital or other health care facility, and this chapter is devoted to those individuals. In this chapter, strategies for planning to become a consultant as a career option are presented, along with some techniques to facilitate the nurse's ability to make the transition from employee to entrepreneur somewhat easier.

CAREER PLANNING

What Is Career Planning?

Career planning, by definition, involves planning for one's progress through life, particularly with regard to progress in a profession or a life's work (Nowak & Grindel, 1984). A *career* differs from a "job." In a job, an individual works primarily for payment, in day-to-day employment. A career, conversely, involves the individual's setting goals and objectives, and following a path that will lead to achievement of those goals.

A career is part of an individual's life roles; those roles include family (spouse, children, and relatives); education; the community; leisure time; and career or work. Emphasis is placed on each of these roles as circumstances change. For example, the nurse who returns to school to obtain an advanced degree is likely to focus more on the role of student (education) than on the role of volunteer (activities in the community). The nurse who has a newborn child may focus on the family role to the exclusion of all others, even the work role.

Occasionally, these life roles conflict with each other. The nurse with a newborn may be distressed at having to return to work to help support the family, and another nurse may be upset because the demands of caring for an elderly parent prevent him or her from returning to college to obtain a master's degree. The well-balanced individual seeks to place nearly equal emphasis on all life roles: finding time for leisure and community activities in addition to fulfilling family and career responsibilities (see chapter 9).

Without career planning, an individual may approach work in an aimless manner, lacking direction and goals. This individual drifts from job to job, perhaps increasing salary or benefits, but never seeming to achieve much in the way of professional advancement. The nurse who plans his or her career, in contrast, seems to be moving ahead and upward with each successive change of position.

Conventional wisdom now suggests that individuals will have as many as four or five careers in a lifetime because of the tremendous and continuous change in the workplace. One of the advantages of the nursing profession is that there are so many options from which to choose, and "new nursing opportunities are constantly emerging" (Kelly & Joel, 1995, p. 670).

Career planning in nursing involves setting goals and objectives, then planning strategies to achieve these goals. Initially, it is necessary to decide what the nurse wants from his or her career. Most nurses want their work to be satisfying, to allow for professional growth, to provide security and belonging, and to reward them for work well done (Swansburg & Swansburg, 1984).

On the basis of these considerations, then, the nurse must decide what is most important. Is it essential to have positions that provide security, or can some risk perhaps be tolerated in exchange for opportunities for professional growth? Thus, the nurse who seeks primarily security may not accept a position as the director of a grant-funded project of 3 years' duration, whereas the nurse who seeks professional growth may gladly move into this position because of the opportunities it affords—not only during the grant period but perhaps afterwards as well.

Hoffman (1984) suggests that the nurse assess the importance of several criteria in relation to work: feelings of self-esteem, security, or accomplishment; opportunities for personal growth and development, independent thought and action; and the sense of helping others. These criteria can be met through a career in nursing—if that career is carefully planned and managed.

Factors in Career Planning: Values, Interests, and Needs

Once the decision has been made about the criteria that must be met by a career, goals can be set. The goals set by the nurse should be both long and short term. Long-term goals will provide incentive to keep striving, whereas short-term goals will provide satisfaction on their attainment— and motivation to continue working to implement long-term goals. Nurses can set career goals by initially assessing where they are and where they desire to be.

Generally, the nurse's goals will be based on the nurse as an individual with values, interests, and needs. Although these elements interact in influencing a nurse's choice of career and the path which that career takes, often the nurse has not explicated them. Explication is necessary in order to understand them and use them effectively in career planning.

Values. Values are those attributes or characteristics that define an individual's behavior. Values are beliefs on which behavior is based; for example, the nurse who values interpersonal relationships may seek a career in psychiatric-mental health nursing, whereas the nurse who values a sense of accomplishment may choose administration as a career. The nurse who loves adventure may choose travel nursing; the nurse who prizes intellectual ability may gravitate toward a career in research.

Interests. Interests are those activities that an individual enjoys—from activities such as cooking and baking to bicycling and skiing or to writing and public speaking. The more that is known about what the nurse likes and finds interesting, challenging, or rewarding, the more likely the individual is to be able to pinpoint possible career paths that will provide opportunities to act on those interests.

One way to identify interests is simply to list them as they come to mind. Once the brainstorming session has been completed, these interests should be converted into the skills they represent: "I like to work with groups in solving problems" may reflect skill in facilitating focus groups, for example. Because individuals do not always see themselves as others see them, however, it is useful to have the skills that the nurse has identified also validated by others. The nurse can prepare a form on which the skills he or she possesses are listed, circulate the list to peers and colleagues, and ask for their candid feedback on the extent to which he or she actually

TABLE 3-1   Interest Assessment Form

Please review the characteristics below and indicate by circling the appropriate choice the extent to which you think these describe me:

	To a great extent				To a minimal extent
I speak well in public. Comments:	5	4	3	2	1
I follow through on instructions. Comments:	5	4	3	2	1
I clarify problems effectively. Comments:	5	4	3	2	1
I am able to delegate to others. Comments:	5	4	3	2	1

possesses those skills. It generally is helpful to provide a scale that the rater can mark, with a space for additional comments; Table 3.1 gives an example.

Responses should be anonymous, to ensure honesty. Responses should be returned for collation to someone other than the nurse if the possibility exists that the nurse could identify the respondent by his or her handwriting. The individual collating these data then provides only a summary of the responses to the nurse and destroys the original forms.

This technique is useful for checking whether one's perceived skills match those observed by others. Discrepancies in the results, if they occur, can be resolved by a second-round questionnaire in which the results are returned to the raters for clarification. In this case, the statement would be made that "Four of five individuals rated my ability to design educational materials for inservice programs that I teach as very low. Please provide specific examples of situations in which that was observed to help me improve my skill in that area. Thank you." If the respondents are confident that their responses will not be conveyed to the nurse, they may be willing to provide additional information that the nurse can use to assess his or her skill. This additional step may be discomforting for the nurse, but it is almost guaranteed to provide helpful information.

Once the information has been gathered and analyzed, the final step is to identify strengths and weaknesses, or areas in which improvement may be needed. Improvement in these characteristics may not be necessary for the nurse to achieve his or her career goals, however, so judgment is needed in deciding how to proceed. If public speaking is not required to accomplish a goal, there may be no purpose in attempting to accumulate experience in making presentations until the need arises.

Needs. Needs are what the individual requires to survive. Needs range from basic survival (e.g., food, air, and water) to higher level needs, such as those identified by Maslow (1970) relating to love and belonging, self-esteem, and self-actualization. Needs are potent forces in determining an individual's behavior. For example, the gap between where an individual currently is and where the individual should be is defined as a learning need (Knowles, 1990). A nurse in a new area of practice—for instance, someone who has moved from acute to home care—generally does not "know the territory" and thus is uncomfortable in the new position. This learning need motivates the individual to close the gap as quickly as possible to reestablish equilibrium and comfort. As a result, the nurse is likely to read home care publications; join organizations, such as the Home Health-care Nurses Association; attend educational meetings on home care topics; and so on—to become more familiar with home health care nursing as rapidly as possible.

Once values, interests, and needs have been assessed, the nurse can use these to identify what is desired and necessary in developing and following a career path. Even though the nurse may be already advanced in a career path, this assessment is useful in determining next steps; career planning is not just for the nurse newly graduated from a school of nursing. The savvy nurse performs a periodic assessment of values, interests, and needs to ensure that he or she stays on an appropriate career path, which may change from time to time.

Using the information gathered about values, needs, interests, and personal characteristics, the nurse then develops career goals. One way to do this is to ask questions, such as the following:

- What do I want to be doing 5 years from now?
- What do I *not* want to be doing 5 years from now?
- What do I see as success in nursing?
- What knowledge and skills do I want 5 years from now?
- What do I want people to say about what I have accomplished?

Responses to these questions generally will incorporate an individual's values, interests, and needs. This information should clearly indicate what the individual wants to do in a chosen career. For example, a response of "to be a consultant on public policy with an international clientele" to the questions "What do I see as success in nursing?" leads to identification of specific activities that must occur for success to be achieved. Responses to these questions should be translated into specific goals; identification of goals is the first step in the process of planning a career.

NURSING OPTIONS

Once the individual's goals have been identified, they are matched with possible options. (At this point, the goals are not translated into long-term and short-term; that step occurs later in the process.)

Careers occur in stages, from initial entry to retirement. A variety of stages between entry and retirement allow flexibility and choice. In fact, such flexibility and choice are among the most attractive attributes of the nursing profession. The nurse may decide in midcareer to change focus, and, indeed, this book is designed to assist the nurse to enter the field of consultation from another area of practice that may be of many years' duration.

A myriad of options exist in nursing that make the nursing profession one of the most exciting in which individuals can work. In its *Forecast 1996* issue, *Money* (Hube, 1995) predicted that the 12 best jobs for the next 12 months would all be in health care. Registered nurse ranked number 5, with an annual salary of $37,000 for positions in nursing homes, home health care, and ambulatory care settings.

There are a variety of ways to describe these and other options for careers in nursing. Swansburg and Swansburg (1984) use clinical practice, education, administration, and research as a framework for describing options in nursing. Henderson and McGettigan (1994) identify "client, setting, nursing functions, nursing roles, health problems, and health professions" as the components to use in analyzing nursing options (p. 124).

Regardless of how the options are analyzed, the first step is obtaining information about them. There are a variety of sources for finding out about nursing options, among them the following:

- People
- Print materials
- Computers

People

People known to the nurse are an excellent source of information about career options. Nurses have many people in their networks who can be a good resource, but often this resource remains untapped. There also are individuals who are currently unknown to the nurse but who can be added to the nurse's networks (see chapter 7) who can provide advice, counsel, and guidance.

Hauter (1993) suggests taking one's boss to lunch and conducting an interview about the boss's career path, what skills and abilities are necessary for his or her job, and what the boss perceives as his or her best qualities.

This information can then be used to plot a career path that is similar to— or completely different from—the boss's. This strategy would work when collecting data from any individuals in a network, not just from bosses.

Collecting data from these individuals should be organized to yield the best results. Haphazard data collection may result in little or no useful information.

Personal interviews are the data-collection method of choice. First, the nurse must identify areas of interest, matching them as closely as possible with the values, interests, needs, and characteristics determined in an earlier step. Next, the nurse must decide what questions to ask . Finally, the nurse must identify the correct person to ask. Perhaps home health care nursing, or research on new and emerging drugs for use in treatment of acquired immuno deficiency syndrome (AIDS), is an area of interest. The nurse would then decide what to ask individuals representing the area of interest. Some possible questions are the following:

1. What are your responsibilities?
2. What do you do in a typical day?
3. What education did you need to prepare for your position?
4. What experience did you need?
5. What do you find satisfying about your work?
6. What do you dislike?
7. What are the opportunities for advancement?
8. What advice do you have for someone seeking a similar position?

These are only a few of the questions that can be asked. Other questions might relate to specifics, such as working in a particular institution, the title of a position, a typical salary range, benefits, and so on.

Once the questions have been decided on, the next step is to identify the individuals in the particular areas of interest to interview. It may be that these individuals are known to the nurse. In the example of home care, the nurse may have colleagues who belong to the district nurses association and who work in home care, and the nurse can interview them. The nurse may go to the library and note the authors of textbooks in home health care nursing, and write or call to set an appointment to interview them. The nurse may make an appointment to interview the director of a home health care agency. The nurse might call the local college or university school of nursing and inquire about faculty members who teach home health care, community, or public health nursing.

In the example of drug research, the nurse may review the literature, particularly that related to clinical trials, and then contact an author for an interview. The nurse may also contact a pharmaceutical company through the local representative to obtain an interview with the appropriate person.

Individuals with a variety of areas of expertise are likely to be members of professional associations, at the state or local level. A good place to contact these individuals is at meetings of districts or chapters of these professional organizations.

Many nursing organizations have subgroups of nurses with a particular area of interest, such as a clinical practice specialty (e.g., intensive care, pediatrics, maternal-child health) or a functional specialty (e.g., staff development, administration, or research). Members of these specialty groups often meet at annual conventions or conferences, and contacts can be made there.

In the event that the individual contacted for the interview is not available, or is not the appropriate person to interview, the nurse can ask for a referral to someone else. It is important to ask for as many referrals to others as possible, to obtain a complete, balanced picture on which to base decisions.

The nurse should always convey thanks for the time and information given. A simple written thank-you note will suffice.

Print Materials

Libraries abound with helpful information. A librarian can help the nurse narrow the search, to save time and energy. An initial visit to the library might concentrate on reviewing current periodicals, such as nursing, medical, and other health care-related journals. Skimming the contents page in each of the publications on display can provide titles of appealing articles. Directories of job opportunities also can provide information and, perhaps more important, a location from which to seek additional information.

Who's Who directories are published in almost every conceivable area. Although individuals are listed in these directories simply by submitting the appropriate information and not necessarily on the basis of merit, nonetheless these directories are good sources to review to find out what people are doing in the areas of research, teaching, publishing, and so on. Directories of professional associations also are a good print source. Listings of consultants also appear in the *Journal of Nursing Administration* (JONA) twice a year.

Computers

The computer provides an avenue to information almost beyond imagination. Connecting to the Internet allows an individual to access services, such as news, sports, and weather; send and receive mail electronically; browse through encyclopedias and dictionaries; obtain financial information; review stock and bond rates; book airline reservations and hotel rooms; play games; and shop through retail stores, catalogs, and discounters.

More relevant to nursing are those computer networks designed by the American Nurses Association (Nurse*Forum) and the American Journal of Nursing Company (AJN Network). Nurse*Forum allows nurses across the country and around the world to network, exchange information and ideas, and share experiences. Efforts are under way to allow specialty nursing associations to develop an area exclusively dedicated to the association, carrying announcements of coming conferences and conventions, press releases, position statements, and new products, among other information.

The AJN Network was initiated under a special projects grant from the Division of Nursing, Department of Health and Human Services. The focus of the network is to provide formal and informal continuing education services to nurses. Services offered on the AJN Network include contact-hour credit offerings; information about patient care; national and international health care news; resource databases, such as a listing of nursing organizations and state boards of nursing; consultation with nurse experts; and a Virtual Conference Center, where users can read abstracts of conference presentations and post messages and questions for the presenters.

Both of these computer networks were relatively new at the time of the writing of this book. It is anticipated that the services offered on these networks will grow as interest in them increases.

Although these—and other—resources are available and are becoming more accessible every day, not everyone avails himself or herself of these new technologies, and nurse consultants are no exception. In the survey of nurse consultants conducted in mid-1995 by the authors, few of the respondents were aware of the existence of the AJN Network (7 of 128, or 5%) and even fewer knew about ANA's Nurse*Forum (5 of 128, or 4%).

These nurse consultants used other forms of technology in their businesses, however. Most (116, or 91%) of the respondents used a personal computer in their consulting practice. Fewer used a facsimile (104, or 81%), and even fewer (68, or 53%) used a computer modem. Although only 35 (27%) were on the Internet, 55 (43%) used e-mail.

It seems fairly certain that computer technology is catching on with nurse consultants and will be an increasingly necessary component of a successful career in consulting. The savvy nurse consultant will attempt to stay apprised of new developments in technology to take advantage of them and thus to maintain a competitive stance in the marketplace.

SETTING CAREER GOALS

Once information has been obtained about possible options in nursing, the nurse sets career goals. These goals should be:

- Both short term and long term
- Stated in order of priority
- Given target dates for completion
- Reviewed periodically

Short- and Long-Term Goals

Career goals should be short term to provide a sense of accomplishment and long term to offer something toward which to strive. Setting only short-term goals will not lead to long range accomplishment or career growth. Conversely, setting only long-term goals with mean that the individual is constantly striving toward some future achievement and feeling no immediate satisfaction, and thus very likely decreasing motivation.

Priority Order

Because individuals have a finite amount of resources (time, energy, and money) to devote to accomplishment of career goals, it is wise to set priorities for these goals so that the most important can be accomplished first. The nurse who sets as a priority establishing visibility in a field of practice might choose first to write for publication or make presentations in an area of expertise rather than setting a goal of obtaining certification. The nurse who wants to demonstrate his or her expertise in a specific area of practice might choose to prepare for certification rather than write for publication.

Target Dates for Completion

Without a specific date for completion of the goal, it will be impossible to determine whether the individual is progressing on his or her career path as planned. The target dates should be realistic and achievable. More time than anticipated should be allotted to achievement of career goals, to allow for the inevitable distractions that may occur. For long-term goals, it may be wise to set interim dates for small steps that lead toward accomplishment of a goal. For example, if the goal is to obtain a doctorate in 5 years, the nurse consultant may set these goals: be enrolled in the program at the end of year 1; have all course work completed by the end of year 3; complete the examination for candidacy by the end of year 4; complete the dissertation by the end of year 5.

Periodic Review

Career goals should be reviewed at least once a year, to be certain that they still are relevant and appropriate. Circumstances in an individual's life may alter career plans and thus should be taken into consideration, because goals may have to be changed. Periodic review of career goals can help the individual refocus energy and serve as motivation for accomplishing his or her goals.

If feasible, the individual should contract with someone, such as a colleague, with similar career goals. Reporting on accomplishments to someone else can serve as a motivating factor for some individuals. Two individuals working together may be able to accomplish some goals more easily than each working alone. For example, studying for a certification examination or writing for publication may be easier when two are working on it than when only one devotes time and energy to the task. Some people, however, prefer to contract with only themselves.

Using the professional goals that have been established to plan a career in nursing takes a great deal of work, but this effort is worthwhile, considering how many years an individual can expect to be in the profession. For example, although the authors have a combined total of 60 years in the profession, if both work until the typical retirement age of 65, they can expect to spend at least 25 more years in nursing.

CAREER MANAGEMENT

Career management requires that the nurse apply strategies and techniques that will facilitate achievement of career goals. Simply stating goals does not ensure that they will be achieved: a great deal of effort must be expended to ensure that the goals are met. Career management involves the following:

1. Identifying, obtaining, and using resources
2. Influencing others
3. Self-development

Identifying, Obtaining, and Using Resources

A variety of resources exist to assist the nurse in achieving career goals. For example, the nurse possesses the resources of basic educational preparation in nursing as well as any advanced degrees, experience in nursing practice, time, energy, and money. Other resources are found in the people who are known by the nurse, in both professional and personal networks. A supportive spouse who cares for the house and children while the nurse goes to school at night is an invaluable resource. A mentor, sponsor, or coach is an excellent example of a "people resource." A scholarship for an advanced degree or a grant for a research project is an example of a financial resource.

Other resources may be less well known and thus not immediately available or accessible to the nurse. Among these resources are knowledge and skill in stress management, time management, negotiation, and conflict resolution, for example.

Influencing Others

Nurses often do not realize how much they influence others. Nurses influence others through their careers by the image they present in a variety of situations: as health care providers; as students, whether in an academic or a continuing education setting; as interviewees for positions. In these situations, and many others, nurses influence not only other individuals but also the institutions in which they are employed—and the nursing profession as well, by their activities.

Self Development

Self-development involves lifelong learning in either academic or continuing education programs. The nurse strives to improve himself or herself personally and professionally through a variety of means: reading the literature and applying the results of research to practice, attending educational events, and getting and staying involved in professional nursing associations through elected and appointed positions.

Career management is not a single activity. Career management involves a variety of activities, such as gathering data, making informed decisions as a result of the data-gathering process, planning strategies, implementing those strategies, and evaluating the results. The process of managing a career is dynamic and changing, as a result of influences from within and without. An example of an internal influence occurs when the nurse experiences dissatisfaction with a position and decides to seek an alternative place of employment. An external influence is one that occurs outside of the nurse: Health care reform and periodic nurse shortages are examples.

BEING SUCCESSFUL

Career management is successful when the individual:

- Is responsible for his or her career decisions
- Takes advantage of opportunities related to career goals
- Implements a plan of action to achieve career goals

- Reassesses progress on achievement of career goals on a regular basis
- Evaluates progress in reaching career goals occasionally

Being successful in managing a career also requires that the individual

- Markets his or her knowledge, skills, and abilities (see chapter 6)
- Cultivates a support network (see chapter 7)
- Rewards himself or herself for achievements
- Develops a trail of experiences and accomplishments that makes him or her unique
- Continuously improves the skills that prepared him or her for nursing
- Learns new skills through participation in continuing education and academic courses; and through other means, such as internships, externships, or mentoring programs

Participation in continuing education programs directly as well as indirectly related to the nurse consultant's area of expertise can expand his or her base of experience and thus make him or her more marketable as a consultant. Expertise in a specialty area is essential for success in consultation. Nurse consultants must maintain and continuously enhance their knowledge and skills in the area or areas in which they consult. Learning skills and abilities outside of the primary area of expertise may help the nurse consultant view his or her practice from a new perspective as well.

It is important first to know the business of consultation as well as the practice area in which the business is founded, but it is also important to expand horizons to other related areas. Learning skills, such as bookkeeping, public relations, marketing, and others, can be of invaluable assistance in growing and developing a nursing consultation business (see chapter 5).

It is equally crucial to success to develop a network that encompasses not only peers within a profession but those outside the profession as well. These contacts can assist with future career moves but also will enhance the nurse consultant's reputation as a respected member of the profession.

In addition to building a series of achievements inside an organization while an employee (e.g., as an internal nurse consultant or intrepreneur) (see chapter 4), perhaps before launching into entrepreneurship, it is important in developing a consulting practice and making contributions to the profession to focus effort on outside activities as well. Work outside the employing organization will enhance an individual's professional image as long as there is no conflict of interest with the primary job. It is unethical—as well as unwise—to devote more energy to outside activities than to one's primary employment. Although it is possible, and even desirable, to freelance and develop a consulting practice during employment that provides security, these outside activities should not detract from the individual's essential work for his or her employer.

Another essential element in preparation for and conduct of consultation activities is that the nurse consultant have a well-prepared curriculum vitae (CV) and résumé. These two documents are developed as a part of career management and kept up to date as the consultant's career proceeds. A curriculum vitae is defined by *Random House Collegiate Dictionary* as "the course of one's life or career." In comparison, a résumé is a chronological account of life experiences, generally for the purpose of obtaining an interview for a specific job.

THE CURRICULUM VITAE

The curriculum vitae or CV is usually designed for the purpose of presenting the educational and experiential qualifications of an individual (Puetz, 1983). The CV is used in a variety of situations: when a potential client is assessing consultants' similar experiences; when an individual is being reviewed for promotion or tenure in an academic setting; when an individual is being introduced before a presentation. The CV also is used in obtaining employment, but generally during the interview—the résumé having served its purpose of generating sufficient interest in the individual to warrant the interview. The CV must be both current and attractive.

Content of the CV

To ensure currency, begin preparing the CV by listing activities and achievements in the following areas:

1. Demographics
2. Education
3. Work experience
4. Honors
5. Research and grants
6. Honors and awards
7. Professional activities
8. Publications

Demographics.   Demographic information includes name, title, place of employment, address, and telephone number. All of this information should be listed at the top of the CV. It is not necessary to add the title "Curriculum Vitae," because a CV has a distinctive "look" and is not likely to be mistaken for anything else. Include with the nurse consultant's name his or her title and current place of employment, and the address of the business. The home address and telephone number are optional but would of course be included if the consultant works from the home. Addresses should include zip codes, and telephone numbers should include area codes.

Additional means of contact, such as fax numbers or e-mail addresses, also should be included on the CV. The telephone number on the CV should be one at which the nurse consultant can be reached during business hours.

It is not necessary to list academic credentials after the name on the CV; these credentials will be included in the section on education. No information on marital status, number of children, state of health, or willingness to relocate appears anywhere on a CV.

Noting the nurse consultant's social security number or Employer Identification Number (EIN) (see chapter 5) on the CV is optional. If, however, the nurse consultant will be paid for services, including the social security number or EIN on the CV may prove a convenience for the client, who does not have to call the consultant for that information when preparing payment.

Education. Completed educational programs are listed on the CV in reverse chronological order, from the most recent to the least recent. List only postsecondary education, specifying the following:

- Institution
- Location
- Degree received
- Year of receipt of degree
- Field of study

Some degrees (PhD and EdD) are commonly known and can be abbreviated. If a degree is not commonly known (ND and DNSc), it should be spelled out and followed by the abbreviation: e.g., nursing doctorate ND.

Only completed educational preparation should be included on the CV. A listing such as "doctoral student" or "doctoral candidate" should be used with caution. Although these terms often are used interchangeably, they reflect different stages of doctoral preparation. A *doctoral student* has been accepted into a doctoral program and is currently completing course work. A *doctoral candidate* generally has completed his or her course work and also has passed the qualifying examinations for admission into candidacy. This error is made innocently but does not reflect well on the integrity of the individual if it appears on the person's CV: It may appear to be an intentional misrepresentation of qualifications because the individual may appear closer to completion of the degree than is actually the case.

It is not necessary, nor is it appropriate, to include attendance at continuing education activities on a CV, because it is expected of a professional that he or she will participate in lifelong learning.

Work Experience.   This section of the CV should include all of the nurse consultant's professional employment in reverse chronological order (the most recent position appears first). Include in the information about employment the following:

- Dates of employment
- Position title
- Institution
- Location

Employment dates should be inclusive of starting and termination dates (e.g., 1983–1989, or March 1983–May 1989).

In the event that a position title is not commonly known, it may be wise to insert a phrase or two to describe the position: for example, care coordinator (nursing unit manager).

Research and Grants.   This section of the CV should list completed or ongoing research. Among the entries should be the nurse consultant's master's thesis and doctoral dissertation. Other research projects that have been completed or are in process as a component of a consultation endeavor should also be listed.

Grant-writing activities also appear in this section, whether or not they were funded, as long as they were approved. Projects that were submitted but not approved for funding should not be listed.

Honors and Awards.   This section of the CV presents the nurse consultant's recognized achievements; including honors that have been awarded. These honors can range from induction into Sigma Theta Tau, the International Honorary Society in Nursing, to acceptance as a fellow of the American Academy of Nursing. Degrees awarded magnum cum laude or summa cum laude should be listed here.

Professional Activities.   This section of the CV includes information on the nurse consultant's current membership in professional organizations. Past memberships should include the dates (e.g., American Evaluation Association 1979–1981). Activity in these organizations, such as elected or appointed positions, should be included as well as the dates these positions were held. Committee activities should be included too. However, the CV should not contain information about civic or community organizations.

This section should also include a listing of professional activities other than memberships, such as teaching, mentoring (e.g., serving on students' thesis or dissertation advisory committees), and consulting. These activities can be grouped under a heading (e.g., accreditation or evaluation) to display an area of expertise.

All of the activities in a specific genre should be listed, but as the CV lengthens, it may be necessary to exercise some selectivity about what items are included. For example, the nurse consultant may list only those presentations given at the state or national level rather than those at the local level.

Publications. The publications section of the CV should list the nurse consultant's publications, such as articles, chapters in books, and entire books. These publications can be listed by types (e.g., books, chapters, and articles).

Publications should be listed consistently, following a style guide, such as the *Publication Manual of the American Psychological Association* (4th ed.). A style guide will ensure accurate listing of authors and other information about each publication.

List publications in reverse chronological order. Publications may be grouped in specific areas of expertise as well (e.g., networking or consultation).

Publications that have been accepted for publication but have not yet appeared in print can be listed as "in press." It is generally not wise to list manuscript submissions that have not yet been accepted for publication, lest the manuscript not be accepted.

In addition to publications in print, publications in other media (e.g., videotapes, computer-assisted instruction, or self-study packets) also can be listed in this section. These types of publications can be listed in subsections of the publications section.

Publications in *Proceedings of Conferences* also can be included here, but those publications that are required as part of an individual's work responsibilities should not be included unless they are important to convey an area of expertise. Thus, an editorial written for an in-house newsletter might not be included unless the topic of the editorial was an area of expertise in which the writer consults.

Additional Points about the CV

To indicate that selectivity was used in listings in the professional activities and publications sections of the CV, these sections can be titled "Selected Professional Activities" and "Selected Publications." This notation will provide a clue that not all possible entries were included. It is important, however, to exclude all entries in a particular category (e.g., contributions to a local newsletter), not merely those that do not reflect well on the nurse consultant, such as a book that was severely criticized in a review or an article that resulted in negative feedback in letters to the editor.

The CV should reflect an individual's professional efforts, but attempting to present a more positive picture than warranted is dishonest.

The CV should be dated. The CV should be updated on a regular basis and each version should carry the date of revision. A good habit to get into is to update the CV on a quarterly basis so that valuable information is not lost, particularly if the nurse consultant is very active professionally.

The CV should be professionally typed, preferably on a computer so that revisions can be made quickly. Storing the CV in a word-processing program means that additions can be made without having to retype pages.

Proofreading the completed CV is essential because typographical errors and misspellings do not reflect well on the nurse consultant. The CV should be printed on good-quality bond paper. Photocopies are acceptable; it is not necessary to always provide an original, but current technology (e.g., laser printers) certainly makes this possible.

THE RÉSUMÉ

The résumé is a document that spotlights or highlights an individual's accomplishments, primarily for the purpose of obtaining a job interview. An effective résumé:

- Matches the employer's needs
- Stands out among a multitude of other résumés
- States qualifications and accomplishments in specific terms
- Is clear and concise (King & Sheldon, 1991)

The résumé should reflect an individual's past accomplishments and potential for future achievements. A résumé, like a CV, must be current and attractive.

Content of the Résumé

The content of the résumé includes the following elements:

- Demographics
- Professional objective
- Experience
- Education
- Personal information
- References

Demographics. As in the CV, demographic information about the individual includes name, title, place of employment, address, and telephone number. Zip codes should be included with addresses and area codes with telephone numbers. This information should be displayed prominently at the top of the résumé. As with the CV, it is not necessary to add the title "résumé," since the résumé too has a distinctive appearance.

Professional Objective. Next, include on the résumé a professional objective. The professional objective is a concise statement of what the individual has to offer a prospective employer, and what the individual wishes to do in his or her career. Some résumé experts, however, suggest that a professional objective may narrow the focus of the job search; they recommend that an objective not be included on a résumé unless the résumé relates only to a specific position, or unless it would be difficult to convey a career goal to a potential employer without an objective statement (King & Sheldon, 1991).

If a professional objective will be included on the résumé, it must be written specifically to relate to a desired position. Computer-generated résumés make this level of specificity possible because a different professional objective can be written for each position for which the individual wishes to apply.

The how-tos of writing a professional objective are described in texts on preparing résumés (Krannich & Banis, 1982, 1995). A simple 4-step process to develop the professional objective is described by Krannich and Banis (1982):

1. Obtain data on skills
2. Corroborate this information
3. Project preferences
4. Test the objective against reality

One method of accomplishing this process was described previously in this chapter (see the section on identifying interests). Skills and abilities can be identified by asking questions such as, "What do I like to do?" "What do I do best?" "What are some activities I don't like to perform?" "What activities have earned me compliments on my performance?" When the skills underlying these activities have been identified (e.g., ability to work with groups; excellent communication skills), they should be corroborated by others. An anonymous questionnaire can be drafted that merely states, "I am trying to validate the skills and abilities I have identified below. Please rate your assessment of the extent to which I possess these skills on a scale of 1 to 5, where 1 is very descriptive of me, and 5 is not at all descriptive of me." Respondents should complete and return the questionnaire without revealing their identify; should there be a chance that the respondent could be identified (by handwriting, for example), a third party should be chosen to collect and collate the responses. Validation of skills and abilities then allows the individual to determine whether he or she is suited for a desired role. This role is identified in the third step of the exercise during which the individual determines a desired role or career and then decides what is necessary to perform that role.

Experience.   This section of the résumé is most closely scrutinized by potential employers. Thus, it is essential to describe these professional experiences in clear, comprehensive terms. Strong words in the active voice (e.g., "managed" rather than "coordinated"; "directed" rather than "assisted") should be used to describe work activities.

Work experiences should be listed in reverse chronological order; the most recent experience appears first. Information to include about work experiences is as follows:

- Dates of employment
- Job title
- Description of responsibilities
- Institution
- Address

Education.   This section follows experience on a résumé because most employers are more interested in a potential candidate's relevant work experience than his or her educational background. Education should be listed in reverse chronological order; additional achievements (graduation magna cum laude or grade-point average) can be emphasized in this section. The description of educational achievements should include the following:

- Degree obtained
- Name of college or university
- Location (city and state)
- Date of graduation

In this section, additional educational accomplishments, such as certification, can be listed, with the name of the certificate and the granting agency as well as the year certification was granted.

Personal Information.   This section should include a statement describing the individual, using data on talents or abilities that distinguish this person from other candidates for the position. These talents or abilities should relate to the desired position and to the individual's professional objective. This personal statement should *not* include information on personal characteristics, such as height and weight, state of health, marital status, or number of children.

References. References included in this section should be specific to the desired position. If the position is in management, references would include those individuals who could attest to the nurse consultant's management expertise. If the consultant is seeking a position in an institution that will involve writing a grant for funding the project, then the references should be those individuals who can verify the nurse consultant's grants-writing expertise.

The names listed as references can actually be added at the time the résumé is prepared. Alternatively, the references section can merely include a statement such as, "References available on request." Then, when the prospective employer requests references, the nurse consultant can submit a separate list of references related specifically to the desired position.

Whether the references are listed on the résumé itself or on a separate page, the information to be included consists of the reference's name, title, employer, address, and telephone number. It is not only common courtesy but absolutely essential for continued relations to request permission before listing someone as a reference. Each time the reference is to be contacted, it is wise to notify him or her of the potential contact, and to coach him or her about the potential position and what should be stressed about the nurse consultant's expertise to ensure a job offer.

Other Information. Other information that can be included on the résumé relates to membership and activities in professional organizations. This information should be included only to the extent that it is related to the professional objective.

Licensure can be included but is not necessary, because an individual is presumed to be licensed in the profession in which he or she is practicing. Nor is it necessary to list participation in continuing education activities, because participation in these is expected of a professional.

Developing a Résumé

A résumé is developed through a three-stage process (Krannich & Banis, 1982; Puetz, 1983). The three steps in the process are the following:

1. Preparation
2. Writing
3. Production

Preparing the Résumé. As with the CV, the résumé should be prepared by the individual. Although there are a number of companies that provide résumé services, most often these résumés all look alike because the company will use a format that works for them. These "boilerplate" formats may not showcase the individual appropriately.

The preparation stage is time-consuming, but the resulting product can be updated and used throughout the individual's career, so the initial time will prove well spent. Updates will not require a great deal of time, but it is wise to review the résumé for needed changes on a routine basis (twice a year, for example).

Writing the Résumé. As with the CV, begin by listing all the data on experience and education. The information collected for the CV can be used on the résumé with a bit of modification. Be certain all the information on work experiences relates to the professional objective.

Ask several colleagues to review the initial draft of the résumé. If a personnel officer is a contact, that individual can also be asked to review the draft. People who employ others can offer useful advise about good and bad résumés—they have seen many of them.

Most résumé experts say the résumé should not be longer than two pages, and preferably only 1 page. "Nice to know" information, such as personal data or names of references, can be deleted to reduce the length of the document to ensure that all of the "need to know" information, such as experience, can be included.

Producing the Résumé. The résumé should be professionally typed. Producing the résumé on a word-processing program facilitates not only initial production but also revisions and updates.

Computer software packages that allow an individual to prepare his or her résumé with a minimum of difficulty can be purchased. Once the résumé information is entered into the program, it can revised or updated easily. Care should be taken, however, that the software will allow the nurse to customize the résumé. Also, the cost of such a program may not be warranted, because most résumés can be produced expeditiously with a word-processing program.

The layout of the résumé is important for eye appeal. Because the purpose of the résumé is to generate interviews, it must stand out from the large number of résumés that will be received for a particular position.

Use plenty of "white space" to set off sections of the résumé. A readable typeface should be used, and the size of the font can be enlarged for section headings. Bold type, italics, and underlining should not be used to highlight sections, because these reduce readability.

The résumé should be proofread several times to ensure that it is grammatically correct, punctuated correctly, and free of typographical errors. The résumé should be printed on high-quality bond paper, preferably with a laser printer but certainly not on a dot matrix printer.

The résumé can be copied for distribution, but good-quality bond paper should be used for any copies. All copies should be perfect; those with streaks or smudges should be discarded.

The individual preparing the résumé should avoid the temptation to use computer graphic programs to add designs. Often these techniques result in a document that is "cute" but hardly professional.

Electronic Résumés. With the advent of computer technology, preparation and distribution of résumés have undergone a revolution, Kennedy and Morrow (1994) and Krannich and Banis (1995) point out that, increasingly, companies interested in hiring individuals are relying on "automated applicant tracking systems" (Kennedy & Morrow, 1994, p. 1), and this requires a completely different résumé from what has been used successfully in the past.

This new approach to hiring requires a résumé that is scannable. The résumé is entered into a computer system either by a large company or by a service bureau whose clients are small companies seeking employees or other human resources, such as consultants.

The computer systems then retrieve potential applicants by keywords in response to an employer's three basic questions (Kennedy & Morrow, 1994, p. 17):

1. Can this person do the job?
2. Will this person do the job?
3. Will this person do the job without stressing out everyone else?

This applicant search eliminates human factors, such as perseverance, resourcefulness, flexibility, organization, or motivation. It also eliminates any positive impression the résumé's appearance might make when viewed by a human. Perhaps worst of all, if a person's résumé is not selected by the tracking system, there is no chance that the individual will be interviewed—and no chance that any problems with the résumé might be overcome during the interview.

Kennedy and Morrow (1994) caution that résumés that may be scanned into an automated applicant tracking system must be prepared with a typeface (e.g., Courier 12 point) that is commonly used and easily readable by scanning software programs. Because these tracking systems rely on keywords, it is equally as important to include "required" and "desired" buzzwords on the résumé as well; these buzzwords are not the "action verbs" recommended above, but rather are nouns that may refer to skills (e.g., accounting or supervision) or to desired companies in which the candidate was previously employed. In the case of a nurse, for example, desired skills—and thus keywords—may be experience in an intensive care unit; familiarity with computers; and a master's degree. These elements would be required buzzwords for which the computer program would search. Desired characteristics may include the ability to speak Spanish, willingness to work the night shift, and supervisory experience.

Kennedy and Morrow (1994, p. 63) offer a list of keywords from a software database that are related to a registered nurse (RN):

Catheter care
Community health care development
Infusion therapy
Peripheral line management
Maternity/child rotation
Acute care
Code 99
Disability management
Intensive care
Postoperative care
Chronic dialysis
Medication administration
Suture removal

Readers will recognize the severely limited description of a nurse's role represented by these keywords. Nonetheless, it is unwise to underestimate the changes that will be caused by technology such as automated applicant tracking systems. If nurses already are being tracked by these systems, albeit on a limited basis, there is no reason to believe that the profession will not be involved to a greater extent in the future.

Kennedy and Morrow (1994) do offer several helpful hints for preparing a résumé that will be computer-friendly.

1. Use a typesize larger than 10-point—12-point or 14-point is best.
2. Do not use italics or underlining; boldface and capitals are acceptable.
3. Do not use graphics or shading.
4. Use lines sparingly.
5. Do not use a dot matrix printer; use a laser printer instead.
6. Always send an original, unfolded, unstapled résumé.

7. Do not use abbreviations or industry jargon.
8. Use a traditional format; print on light-colored paper.
9. Place the individual's name first on the résumé, above any other information.
10. If the résumé is to be faxed, use a "fine" rather than "standard" setting to enhance readability.

These hints can be followed when sending a résumé to a company that is likely to use an automated applicant tracking system or is a client of a service bureau that uses such a system. It is incumbent for the nurse consultant to avail himself or herself of any means to spread the word about his or her consulting services, even those that seem to be focused on finding potential employers. A potential employer can be converted into a client for consulting services if the nurse consultant's expertise matches what is being looked for by the employer.

Employers will appreciate the opportunity to obtain services for a fixed fee that does not involve paying benefits. The nurse consultant should use this as a bargaining point. A previous employer, if satisfied with the nurse consultant's performance as an employee, is more likely to agree to give the nurse consultant the opportunity to show what he or she can do than a client who is not familiar with the nurse consultant's previous work.

SUMMARY

In this chapter, the focus has been on developing career plans. The career that is planned should be based on all available information, and on informed decisions about the match between skills and abilities and the potential career path. Once a career path is chosen, goals and objectives should be set to serve as a road map to establish direction. Then, periodic assessment of progress occurs to ensure that movement is being made toward the established goals.

Tools such as a curriculum vitae and a résumé are necessary in career planning and management. These documents can easily be prepared by the nurse consultant to showcase his or her accomplishments.

Moving from an employment setting to a consulting business is not an easy step, but will be less problematic if the nurse consultant is prepared to plan for the move and implement strategies to ensure success. Planning a career path and managing that career not only will result in achievement of the career goals that were set, but also will ensure that the nurse consultant reaches a phase in his or her career that will generate a great deal of satisfaction as well as contributions to the profession.

REFERENCES

Hauter, J. (1993). *The smart woman's guide to career success.* Hawthorne, NJ: Career Press.

Henderson, F. C., & McGettigan, B. O. (1994). *Managing your career in nursing.* New York: National League for Nursing Press.

Hoffman, V. R. (1984). *New directions for the professional nurse.* New York: Arco.

Hube, K. (1995, December). Where the jobs will be in '96 (hint: think healthy). *Money/Forecast 1996, 24,* 21–22, 24.

Kelly, L. Y., & Joel, L. A. (1995). *Dimensions of professional nursing* (7th ed.). New York: McGraw-Hill.

Kennedy, J. L., & Morrow, T. J. (1994). *Electronic resume revolution.* New York: John Wiley & Sons.

King, J. A., & Sheldon, B. (1991). *The smart woman's guide to resumes and job hunting.* Hawthorne, NJ: Career Press.

Knowles, M. S. (1990). *The adult learner: A neglected species* (4th ed.). Houston, TX: Gulf.

Krannich, R. L., & Banis, W. J. (1982). *High impact resumes & letters.* Chesapeake, VA: Progressive Concepts.

Krannich, R. L., & Banis, W. J. (1995). *High impact resumes and letters* (6th ed.). Manassas Park, VA: Impact.

Maslow, A. (1970). *Motivation and personality* (2nd ed.). New York: Harper & Row.

Nowak, J. B., & Grindel, C. G. (1984). *Career planning in nursing.* Philadelphia: Lippincott.

Puetz, B. E. (1983). *Networking for nurses.* Rockville, MD: Aspen.

Swansburg, R. C., & Swansburg, P. W. (1984). *Strategic career planning and development for nurses.* Rockville, MD: Aspen.

4

The Internal
Nurse Consultant

Although much of this book is targeted toward entrepreneurial nurse consultants, there is a burgeoning role for nurse consultants within agencies or institutions. This chapter is devoted to those who aspire to consult within their employing organization and to those who are already fulfilling the role of internal adviser, coach, confidant, teacher, and problem solver.

DEFINITIONS

Internal Consultants

An internal nurse consultant is one who provides advice, guidance, or counsel within an employment setting. The internal nurse consultant is usually an employee and may have long been involved with the agency or institution; this individual has a set of skills or a knowledge base that is unique and in demand across several units or facilities within an organization. The internal nurse consultant frequently has a dual role within the employment setting—for example, as an oncology clinical nurse specialist and pain management consultant, or as an employee health nurse and a consultant on industrial safety and health.

Lange (1987) describes the internal consultant as a "person existing within an organization who is given the responsibility to plan and implement constructive change as an identifiable formal or informal function" (p. 15).

Block (1981) suggests that any time a person is in a position to give advice to another, that person is acting as a consultant. Such a definition suggests that many employees are consultants. For the purposes of this chapter, the internal nurse consultant will be defined as a nurse who has purposefully assumed the role of consultant within the employing agency.

Intrapreneurs

In the last 10 years, several classic studies have been written about intra-preneurs. Pinchot (1985), who coined the word "intrapreneurship," defines an intrapreneur as an employee who is innovative, creative, and willing to take risks in the work setting by forging ahead with a new product, idea, or process. The intrapreneur works long hours, may have ideas or inventions that are at first discounted, and may be rejected or ridiculed repeatedly. Roadblocks can confront an intrapreneur who is trying to bring fresh, different, or unusual approaches to "the way we do business around here." Despite obstacles, intraprenuers are so driven that they push forward with a new notion regardless of the odds and their opponents.

Manion, a registered nurse, has written about nurse intrapreneurs. Manion (1990) defines a nurse intrapreneur as "one who creates innovation within the health care organization through the introduction of a new product, a different service, or simply a new way of doing something" (p. 2). Manion (1994) suggests that the nurse intrapreneur has a healthy curiosity, is always on the lookout for how something might be done differently, takes responsibility for his or her work, is a good listener, and is able to sell ideas to others. Both Pinchot (1985) and Manion (1990) report that the intrapreneur has a vision of what the world "could be like" and an incessant passion, daring, and drive to make that vision happen.

Manion (1994) has recorded the efforts and results of numbers of nurse intrapreneurs. For example, she reports on a nurse who created a board game for the review of code procedures that is now marketed nationwide. She recounts the story of the Vermont operating room nurse who almost single-handedly secured state funding to test ideas on waste recycling and is now coordinating waste recycling efforts across the institution.

Although an internal consultant may not necessarily be an intrapreneur, the authors suspect that many internal consultants got their start providing advice or counsel across the organization because they had a novel approach to patient care, an unusual strategy for improving a delivery mechanism or system or a nagging notion that "there is a better way to do this"; and because they kept digging for the better way, and when they could not find one, they invented it. In addition to inventing the "better mousetrap," many of those intrapreneurs provide advice and counsel on its use and its continuous improvement.

This chapter focuses on the internal nurse consultant: an employee with special expertise or a special set of skills who is called on to provide advice across the employing agency. However, there are many other applications for the nurse intrapreneur—the nurse employee who is constantly experimenting, inventing, and challenging the status quo. As we move into an age of creativity, one that demands the constant acquisition of new knowledge and skills, the authors hope this chapter will inspire more nurses to assume the roles of internal consultant and intrapreneur.

SKILLS OF THE INTERNAL CONSULTANT

The *skill set* for the internal nurse consultant is comparable to that of the external consultant. Attributes of the consultant have been addressed in chapter 1. Special emphasis on the following traits is important for the internal consultant:

- Communications skills
- Problem-solving skills
- Nursing knowledge or "product skills"
- Process skills
- "Can do" attitude

Communications Skills

Champy (1995) reports that the best leaders in an organization are the best communicators. Further, Champy notes that the best communicators are the ones who deliver a forceful message to employees that the employees accept and act on. In many respects, the same can be said for the internal nurse consultant. The successful internal nurse consultant will be a communicator with a message that people accept and act on.

It is likely that the internal nurse consultant will be continuously challenged to get people to listen or act on her or his ideas or thoughts on a particular problem. As Lange (1987) suggests, the internal consultant might be viewed as part of the problem rather than as an adviser with an idea or solution.

Whether imparting new knowledge, advising on building skills, or devising strategies for change, the internal nurse consultant must be a consummate listener, a credible persuader, and a forceful communicator. Special attention to developing and using public speaking and presentation skills will also help the internal nurse consultant address a variety of audiences.

Problem-Solving Skills

The internal nurse consultant will be challenged to stay focused on a particular problem or task. As Lange (1987) points out, the internal nurse consultant may act in dual roles. The nurse might be both a consultant and a clinical nurse specialist with a patient caseload. Thus, it might be easy to get caught up in caring for a patient population and spend less time on the consulting assignment.

The internal consultant is likely to confront consulting assignments that necessitate working intraunit or interunit. Thus, the ability to solve problems on a small and large scale is important. Orsburn, Moran, Musselwhite, and Zenger (1990) report that a simple, easy-to-use problem-solving process that helps people is best. The problem-solving process they recommend calls for

- Identifying the problem
- Deciding on the cause or causes
- Selecting a solution
- Implementing the solution
- Following up

Although the external consultant often provides recommendations and then leaves an organization, the internal consultant makes recommendations and remains in the agency after advice is given and, therefore, will be challenged to implement the advice supplied.

Nursing Knowledge or "Product Skills"

The internal nurse consultant must have and maintain cutting-edge knowledge in the practice area in which the consultation is offered. The external consultant who has clients across a variety of clinical settings will have continuing exposure to varied approaches, knowledge, and ways of work. Special effort must be made by the internal nurse consultant to reach beyond the employing institution to keep abreast of what others are doing and then bring that new knowledge to the employment setting. The internal nurse consultant can also take advantage of the knowledge and skills that inside colleagues possess and synthesize to share across the organization.

The internal consultant may want to achieve a designation, such as certification or an advanced practice credential, that attests to expertise in practice or acquisition of knowledge. Such external recognition is one way to affirm the consultant's knowledge and skills internally.

Process Skills

Despite all the management literature and advice to the contrary, many health care organizations remain hierarchical and bureaucratic. The internal consultant, by virtue of employment status, will be a part of an organization's hierarchy and will probably have to manipulate the bureaucracy to get ideas heard. On the other hand, the internal nurse consultant's knowledge of processes and politics within an institution should assist in getting ideas implemented. The internal consultant's familiarity with internal systems will inform recommendations and enable suggestions and advice to be customized to mesh with the values, culture, and work systems of the agency.

The internal consultant will need a good set of facilitation skills, including proficiency in meeting management, dexterity in writing reports, adeptness in bridging management layers and social strata, deftness in persuading fellow employees to another viewpoint, and dexterity in resolving conflicts.

"Can Do" Attitude

Whereas the external consultant might be motivated by building and maintaining a client base, money, independence, and the sense of being one's own boss, the internal consultant is likely to find it more difficult to remain motivated. Organizational bureaucracies, politics, and rules can make it difficult to be enthusiastic about providing advice or trying to bring about change. Nevertheless, enthusiasm for one's work and confidence in one's abilities can go a long way toward maintaining a "can do" attitude. An understanding of human nature and the process of change is also an important component of the internal consultant's tool kit.

The internal consultant might find it helpful to reach out to other internal consultants in the agency or community for support. Local chapters of professional associations, graduate nursing programs, honorary nursing societies, and alumni associations can also be good forums for support, exchange of information, and ideas.

PROS AND CONS OF INTERNAL CONSULTING

There are advantages and disadvantages to being an internal consultant.

Pros

The advantages are the following:

- Status as an employee
- Knowledge of the workplace
- Network of colleagues
- Support systems

Employee Status.   Status as an employee carries with it cash compensation on a regular basis; benefits, such as health insurance, life insurance, and a retirement plan; paid time off for vacation, sick leave, or bereavement; tuition reimbursement; and on-the-job education, training, and development. Federal and state taxes are routinely deducted from the internal nurse consultant's paycheck. Employment status may provide the opportunity for organizational advancement, status, or position. In contrast, the external nurse consultant who is not an employee will have to provide his or her own benefits, such as health insurance, and pay taxes quarterly. The external consultant often finds that cash compensation is irregular and may fluctuate from month to month. In addition, the external consultant will have to reach out to the broader community to obtain additional education and develop and maintain networks. The internal nurse consultant does not have to put his or her own funds at risk, such as financing business start-up costs, as the entrepreneurial consultant does. Further, the internal consultant's employer may be willing to provide capital for new products or services that the internal consultant might suggest or design, whereas the external consultant may have to look for investors or borrow money.

Workplace Knowledge.   The internal consultant will have knowledge of the institution's policies, procedures, and processes. The agency's vision, mission, goals, culture, and values will be familiar to the internal nurse consultant, who will therefore not have to spend valuable time learning about these matters before embarking on a consulting assignment. The organization's strengths and weaknesses will be known to the internal consultant, as will ongoing opportunities for matching the consultant's skills to the organization's needs. By contrast, the external consultant must spend time becoming familiar with the institution's mission, objectives, and ways of working.

Colleague Networks.   The internal nurse consultant will have a ready-made network of nurse colleagues and associates in other disciplines to call on for guidance, tips, or information. One of the frequent laments of the external nurse consultant is the lack of regular contact with colleagues for generating ideas and sharing information. The internal nurse consultant is likely to be familiar with the strengths and weaknesses of people in his or her network and can draw on the talents of others as needed for a particular assignment.

Support Systems.   The internal nurse consultant will have access to computer systems; informational databases; libraries; copiers; faxes; and, most likely, clerical support. Although the internal nurse consultant is accountable and responsible for his or her actions, the employer assumes some of the risk as well. The external consultant usually has all risk and accountability for decisions made and actions taken.

Cons

The disadvantages of being an internal consultant are several. Drawbacks can include the following:

- Bosses
- Roles
- Compensation
- Risk
- Effectiveness
- Biases

Bosses. The internal nurse consultant will probably report to a "boss" and therefore will have to meet the expectations and rules imposed by the supervisor and the employing agency. For example, hours of work may be prescribed or attendance at meetings required. Block (1981) suggests that saying no to one's manager can be difficult for the internal consultant, who will very likely have to respond to his or her own manager's needs and wants as well as those of the manager's manager. Further, Block suggests that the consultant may be asked to sell his or her own department's approach to an issue or problem rather than use his or her best judgment as to how an issue or problem might be tackled.

Pinchot (1985) suggests that the intrapreneur find an internal sponsor for support and help in dealing with the politics and processes of a bureaucracy. The internal nurse consultant might also find an internal sponsor helpful in building and sustaining an internal consulting practice. Such a sponsor should be someone who is familiar with the agency, has credibility across the company, and is able to manage the political system and guide the internal consultant through the inevitable shoals of the organization's culture and ways of working.

Roles. Frequently, the internal nurse consultant will have one or more roles related to patient care, as staff development educator or shift supervisor. Multiple roles can lead to limited time to pursue consulting activities and to confusion among coworkers as to the part being played. Lange (1987) points out that the internal consultant can be thrust into the role of manager or supervisor, and that such line responsibility connotes authority or power over others that is clearly at odds with the role of consultant or adviser. Block (1981) notes that the internal consultant has a job level in the organization that is widely known, and this level can limit influence and access to key people in the organization.

Compensation. The internal consultant will most likely be paid according to the compensation plan of the employing institution. Opportunities for additional compensation may be limited to annual adjustments in the salary scale or cost-of-living increases. Additional duties, such as providing counsel and advice across the organization, may not result in additional compensation for the internal nurse consultant. Health care organizations, particularly nonprofit groups, have been slow to devise incentive plans or programs that award more compensation for the assumption of additional duties or in recognition of innovation or risk taking. Profit sharing has been anathema in many health care circles.

Risk. Organizational bureaucracy and hierarchy can make it difficult for the internal nurse consultant to venture into new areas of practice or ways of working. Innovation can be thwarted by recalcitrant employees, reluctant superiors, or limiting policies and regulations. The lengthy time for approval of new ideas or approaches may result in missed opportunities or such dilution of goals that the work of the internal consultant is considered ineffective.

Effectiveness. The internal consultant can be perceived as part of the problem rather than part of the solution. Lange (1987) notes the internal consultant might get by with average performance. Mediocre performance is more likely to be tolerated with an internal consultant than with an external consultant—who has to prove competence repeatedly to stay in business. In addition, responsibilities to the employer other than the consulting role can hamper productivity and effectiveness. Also, external advisers are often viewed as having greater credibility or more expertise than those employed in an organization. It has long been observed that "a prophet is not without honor, save in his own country."

Block (1981) remarks that if the internal consultant makes an error on a job, everyone will know it. Such disasters might be tolerated a time or two, and then the demand for services will decrease, leaving the internal consultant to return to a former job, or worse, unemployed and with no other client base.

Another problem is that an agency or its employees can become dependent on the internal consultant. Day-to-day access to an internal nurse consultant can lead to relying on the consultant to implement recommendations rather than working with the consultant as coach, adviser, teacher of a new set of skills, or bearer of new knowledge.

Biases. The internal nurse consultant is not immune to organizational proclivities. Such predispositions might include having favorite coworkers or managers or preferred ways of working, or being committed to methods previously designed by the internal consultant when working in another role or to ways of work suggested by another internal or external consultant. Also, the internal nurse consultant might have a reputation marred by previous disagreements with coworkers or might hold a grudge after being passed over for a particular assignment. On the other hand, the internal consultant, having been singled out by management for the role of adviser, counselor, or confidant, might be perceived as a "fair-haired child."

GETTING STARTED AS AN INTERNAL CONSULTANT

Becoming an internal consultant can happen by design or default. The authors posit that most internal nurse consultants have "fallen" into the role through proposing an idea or innovation that led naturally to teaching, telling, or conferring with a colleague or group of fellow employees. As hospitals, schools of nursing, industries, and others struggle to survive in today's marketplace, the health care field is fertile ground for the design and implementation of an internal consulting practice for the registered nurse. Table 4.1 illustrates some questions to help an individual decide whether he or she has the aptitude necessary to be an internal consultant.

The steps for development of an internal consulting practice are not unlike the steps for creating an external practice:

1. A need must be identified within the employing agency.
2. The consultant must have the skills to match the need.
3. The consultant must be able to sell or market his or her skills to those in need.
4. Those in need must retain the person with the skill set to solve the problem or manage the issue.

Need

Necessity has been described as the mother of invention. A look around the employment setting will usually result in identification of a myriad of problems that need solving or issues that need attention. The internal nurse consultant should be alert for opportunities to use skills beyond the particular job for which he or she was employed. Once a problem or need is identified, the aspiring internal consultant should ask the following questions:

- What is the problem that needs to be solved or the issue that needs to be tackled?
- Is this a new or an old problem or issue?
- Are others concerned about this matter?

TABLE 4.1   **Internal Consultant: Do You Have What It Takes?**

Yes	No	
___	___	Do you have skills or knowledge that should be used more broadly within the organization?
___	___	Are you called on frequently to provide advice to colleagues, peers, or other health professionals within your agency?
___	___	Are you constantly exploring new ways of doing things?
___	___	Do you mix easily with people with a variety of skills, viewpoints, and educational backgrounds?
___	___	Are you always on the lookout for a way to test or evaluate your ideas or knowledge?
___	___	Are you constantly looking for new knowledge and skills?
___	___	Do you love to work (i.e., do not mind long hours, weekends, holidays, or returning to the clinical area or office after you have gone home)?
___	___	Are you good at persuading others to take your view point?
___	___	Do you have good listening skills (i.e., really hear what is being said to or around you)?
___	___	Do you have good writing skills (i.e., convey thoughts clearly, succinctly, and enthusiastically)?
___	___	In the face of rejection, can you pick yourself up and start over again?
___	___	Do you like to teach?
___	___	Are you patient (i.e., do not mind repeating what you have just explained or demonstrated, are willing to look for different ways to convey an idea, and think no question is dumb)?

Note. If you answered "yes" to each of these questions, you may want to explore how you might consult within your organization.

Skills

Given a clear identification of the need, the prospective internal nurse consultant should ask the following questions:

- What do I know about this matter?
- Do I have knowledge, expertise, or an idea that should be contributed to this subject?
- Am I interested in working on the problem or issue?
- Have I dealt with a similar situation? Can I apply what was learned from that experience to this situation?
- Do I have any biases, conflicts, or previous experience that would interfere with consulting on this issue?

- Has another consultant, internal or external, addressed this matter previously? What were the results?

If the prospective consultant decides to match his or her skills to the need, the nurse should take a piece of paper and write the problem or issue down in his or her own words. Describe the matter thoroughly. Make any inquiries necessary to enhance understanding and refine the written document.

Next, the consultant should match his or her skills to the need, preferably on the same paper on which the problem or issue has been described. For example, the issue might be a need to clarify the mission and focus of the school of nursing for the next 3 to 5 years. This need might be matched to the internal nurse consultant's skills in group facilitation and strategic planning. After the aspiring consultant matches the need of the school with his or her skills, he or she sets the document aside for a day or two. Then the consultant picks up the document again and makes any refinements necessary. If the consultant is still convinced that his or her skills match the need, a trusted mentor or coach might be contacted to talk the matter through. To get an unbiased, objective viewpoint, it is best to seek an adviser with no ties to the prospective consultant's employer. Take those suggestions deemed appropriate and refine the "needs-skills" document.

Marketing and Making the Sale

Now that the budding internal consultant has spotted a problem and matched his or her skill set to tackling the matter, it is time to market or sell his or her services. The key is to have the right solution to the right problem at the right time. At the time of the writing of this book, health care institutions are becoming increasingly competitive. They are interested in becoming more efficient and more cost-effective, saving money, earning money, employing fewer people, and improving the quality of products and services delivered. So this is an opportune time for solutions that offer these benefits.

Manion (1990) suggests that most innovations will be successful when backed by an interested, enthusiastic team of coworkers. Thus, the aspiring internal consultant might identify a few people who are interested in the issue or problem, get their views on the matter, and see if they have any ideas for a solution, change, or response. The internal consultant should not impose a ready-made solution on the group; rather, the consultant should search for others' ideas, options, and opinions. The nurse consultant may want to share potential approaches to the problem and ask for pros, cons, or other ideas. Dissidents should be as welcome to the process as supporters. Team members whose skills supplement those of the consultant should be sought.

Another consideration at this time is the support of the organization's managers and administrators. Many employing agencies are still extraordinarily hierarchical, and this means that the need and the nurse consultant's ability to deal with the need must be presented to the immediate supervisor. The internal consultant should seek time with the supervisor to make a case for dealing with the problem. A "sale" to the consultant's manager is most likely to be made if the consultant can point out benefits to the manager. The wise consultant will have considered how dealing with the matter will position the manager within the organization (i.e., the manager will look good for having contributed to solving a problem, resolving an issue, or providing an innovation to the organization). The goal is to get the solution or idea to the final decision maker. The consultant might then enlist the supervisor to get support further up the management ladder, to the point where the ultimate decision can be made.

In organizations where lines of authority are less important to day-to-day operation, the nurse consultant might go directly to the decision maker. In this instance, the consultant will want to describe the need clearly, and his or her skills for dealing with the need. Part of the sales pitch might include asking for the ideas or input of the decision maker while persuading the decision maker to retain the consultant.

Depending on the type of consulting services the aspiring internal consultant seeks to provide, the development of a business plan may be appropriate (see chapter 5).

FORMALITIES

Agreements

Once the internal sale is made, it is time to determine whether an oral agreement about the work to be done will suffice or if a written agreement is preferable. Manion (1990) suggests that the scope of a project may determine the necessity for a written agreement. A written agreement can define the project, clarify the scope of work, address the time lines involved, clarify ownership of any new products or inventions, and address the resources the organization is willing to commit to the work, including any special compensation of the internal consultant. Although the internal consultant has every right to ask for an agreement in writing, some employing organizations will be reluctant to enter into a written special agreement with an employee, preferring an oral arrangement for the work to be done. There is no one right answer for every situation. The internal consultant will have to weigh and measure the work and the risk involved. If there is a new product or innovation involved, such as a treatment modality, the issue of patent or copyright (see below) is likely to arise. If a new medical device is created or publication prepared, the question of royalties may arise. For example, the issue may be what percentage of royalty the employer receives and what percentages the consultant receives. These matters generally should be resolved in writing.

The employer will often take the position that the internal consultant as an employee, has produced the invention on company time and with company resources. The consultant, on the other hand, may contend that the creativity and experimentation that led to the innovation occurred during nonwork hours. To avoid misunderstandings, hard feelings, and even litigation, all parties are wise to put their agreements in writing. Manion (1990) reports that many managers will appreciate the intrapreneur's preparation of a written document containing key points of the agreement.

It is at this stage that lawyers may get involved. The employer may want the corporate attorney to review any agreement to be entered into with an employee for consulting services. The employee may feel the need for counsel as well. Consideration should be given to any employment policies that might apply to the situation, and to any precedents.

Another consideration in getting an agreement for internal consultation is whether or not there is a collective bargaining agreement that stipulates who does what work in the facility. The internal nurse consultant may be a part of the bargaining unit and may thus be constrained by the contract. Any contractual arrangement between an institution and a group of its employees should be checked for applicability to the internal nurse consultant irrespective of the consultant's inclusion in the bargaining unit.

Compensation

Compensation is often thought of as cash paid for work done. In fact, compensation can include cash; benefits, such as health or life insurance; time off; perquisites, such as membership in a health club; or recognition, such as awards. The internal nurse consultant will no doubt be compensated for work as an employee of the hospital or institution. The consultant and employer may concur that additional compensation of some sort is appropriate for the consultation provided. As Manion (1990) suggests, if there is no direct financial reward or increased revenue as a result of an innovation or, in the case of the internal adviser, consultation provided, the issue of compensation may not arise. However, if additional revenue accrues to the institution, or significant cost reductions are achieved or significant hours are spent by the internal consultant on a project, it is appropriate to consider additional compensation.

The compensation can be awarded in several ways. Cash can be bestowed on the consultant. Perhaps a percentage of revenue earned or expenses saved will be awarded. In some agencies, the consultant's department will acquire a portion of any cost savings or revenue to be applied to unit activities such as staff development, or to the acquisition of additional resources, such as more computers, upgrades of software, or remodeling of an employee lounge.

Noncash recognition can be bestowed on the consultant or intrapreneur's department. This recognition can take the form of a feature article in the facility's bulletin, a reserved parking spot in the hospital garage, a trip to a professional seminar or an association meeting, or an opportunity to extend consulting services to other departments or facilities within the corporate family. Extra time off might also be given to the internal nurse consultant. Noncash benefits may have personal tax implications. Benefits such as time off may be influenced by wage and hour laws. Thus, careful records of all compensation should be kept, and personal tax or financial advisers consulted as appropriate.

A continuing informal survey by one of the authors reveals that most employees find the opportunity for decision making to be one of the greatest job motivators. The internal nurse consultant might find that the additional responsibilities that go with innovation, risk taking, and decision are ample recognition for consulting work.

Intrapreneurs and internal consultants should not be afraid to raise the issue of recognition and remuneration for work done, innovations developed, or consultation provided. Along with raising the issue, the consultant may want to provide several options for recompense along with any data that demonstrate cost savings achieved or revenue generated.

Copyrights, Trademarks, and Patents

One of the risks an internal consultant takes is that an idea or innovation will be taken and implemented by another person. As Manion (1990) notes, it is not possible to patent ideas, but it is possible to protect products or processes. Although a product or process is not likely to be taken from the internal consultant, it is prudent to assess the risk and determine if the work should be legally protected. Such protection might come in the form of a patent, copyright, or trademark.

A patent is granted by the federal government subsequent to a long, arduous process of form filing, research, and payment of a fee. A patent can be obtained for a tangible innovative product. A patent does not apply to ideas, processes, or written material. Manion (1990) writes that the best protection for many products is to produce them quickly and gain recognition and support from customers. Such support might be gained through demonstrating how an innovation makes giving patient care easier or more efficient. Recognition might be achieved through testing an innovation with those most likely to be affected, and changing the product or process according to test results.

A literary work, such as this book, can be protected by copyright. A copyright is granted by the U.S. Copyright Office subsequent to submission of the work to be copyrighted, completion of an application, and payment of a fee. As Manion (1990) reports, copyrighting is not well understood. There is often confusion as to who owns the copyright on work done for hire—for example, a manual created by the internal nurse consultant on pain management. Does the nurse own the copyright by virtue of creating the document, or does the employer own the document because the internal nurse consultant is an employee? Ownership should be discussed by the nurse and employer, and the agreement reached should be put in writing.

A trademark protects an organization's name, logo, or symbol. Trademarks are issued by the U.S. Department of Commerce subsequent to completion of an application, submission of the material to be trademarked, payment of a fee, and a search to ensure that the name, logo, or symbol, or some variation thereof, is not otherwise trademarked.

The intrapreneur should clarify at the outset the ownership of products, literary works, symbols, or names. Is the owner the nurse intrapreneur or the employing agency? In some instances, joint ownership of material can be arranged.

In addition, the internal nurse consultant will want to ensure that creations such as an educational curriculum, a training strategy, a novel treatment, or a medical device can be used by the nurse on leaving the employing institution. The authors have heard many stories from nurses who developed workshops, manuals, or medical devices only to be denied permission to take the creation outside the institution. Ownership of products created by the internal consultant and use of the products if the nurse is no longer employed by the institution should be clarified at the outset, before the work is started. Agreements or understandings between the employer and nurse consultant should be put in writing and signed by both parties.

ISSUES FOR THE INTERNAL CONSULTANT

Confidentiality

As noted elsewhere, keeping clients' confidences is one of the major rules of the nursing and consulting professions. As Lange (1987) asserts, access to people and information is integral to the consultant's job and is required for effective intervention by the consultant. Thus, the consultant is often privy to information about others and the recipient of personal confidences.

For the internal consultant, the matter of confidentiality will be overlaid with the issue of trust (i.e., trust in the internal nurse consultant). Trust is belief in and certainty about another. For the internal nurse consultant, reputation, relationships with coworkers, and perceptions of competence will influence how she or he is viewed—that is, whether there is belief in and certainty about the consultant as a nurse and person. Trust will precede the imparting of confidences, particularly secrets.

The internal nurse consultant will find keeping confidences a particular challenge. Most institutions have an active grapevine, which carries information without regard to its accuracy. Although the nurse consultant may not purposefully participate in the organization's grapevine, the work of the consultant may be carried on the grapevine and may be subject to repetition, speculation, and distortion. The internal consultant's supervisor or other superiors may expect information to be shared that the consultant believes is proprietary or that was given in confidence.

The best way to handle the issue of confidences in the workplace is to deal with the matter directly with one's manager and internal clients at the outset of the consultation. What information can be shared and what will be held in confidence should be clarified initially. Special situations will arise that must be handled on a case-by-case basis. The internal nurse consultant will do the best work with the trust and confidence of all with whom he or she interacts and on whom the project relies.

The internal nurse consultant will have daily access to networks of friends, colleagues, and coworkers with whom he or she might be particularly close. Care should be taken not to share information with the admonishment that it should be kept in confidence (it will not be) or to divulge data carelessly in an unguarded moment. One slip can ruin the internal nurse consultant's business and reputation.

Ethical considerations—such as honesty, use of judgment, maintenance of competence, and dignity of behavior (outlined in chapter 8)—are as important for the internal consultant as for the external consultant.

Working With Other Consultants

From time to time, the internal consultant will need assistance from one or more consultants external to the organization or will be placed in a position of working with external consultants selected by other departments or other internal consultants. Lange (1987) calls this "collaborative internal-external consultation."

Such internal-external consultation is increasingly prevalent as institutions downsize and outsource work. Outsourcing is a popular way to obtain staff; work on special projects such as the development of critical pathways; or provide training, and obtain some computer hardware and software. As hospitals and other health care agencies are acquired by or are merged with other groups, working with consultants from other parts of the corporation becomes more likely. Although such consultants are internal to the corporate structure, any particular consultant may be external to the department or facility for which the internal nurse consultant works. Thus, the collaborative internal-external model of consultation, or even a collaborative internal-internal model, is likely to become more prevalent.

Lange (1987) reports that a good approach to matching an internal and external consultant is for the internal consultant to participate in selecting the external consultant. The same advice applies to internal-internal consultant matches. The internal consultant should

- Be clear about the project to be undertaken
- Identify skills that must be obtained externally and that complement the internal consultant's skills
- Be sure superiors support the idea of retaining an external consultant
- Ensure that superiors and the internal consultant agree on the role of the external consultant
- Interview external candidates, seeking a reciprocal personality, good communication skills, and good "people skills"
- Seek a person willing to collaborate with the internal consultant

Once an external consultant has been obtained, the internal consultant will want to

- Affirm the role and tasks of the external consultant, preferably in writing, along with any special arrangements agreed to, such as office space and access to records or files
- Take the lead in working with the external adviser in developing a work plan that details the project, the responsibilities of the internal and external consultant, and time lines
- Establish a routine communication link with the external consultant for exchange of information, clarification or resolution of issues or problems that arise, review of work in progress, and adherence to time lines
- Introduce the external consultant to staff and managers

As Lange (1987) notes, the relationship between an internal and an external consultant can be competitive and difficult. The internal consultant can feel threatened and undermined. The external consultant can feel confused and adrift. Either consultant by virtue of his or her position can feel superior to the other. Attention to development of a collaborative working relationship at the outset can go a long way to ward off such difficulties. The internal consultant's participation in selecting an external consultant increases the chance of a truly collaborative, mutually beneficial effort.

It is possible that the internal consultant will not have a say in the selection of an external consultant. Such an situation can make it difficult for the internal consultant to work with the external consultant. The internal consultant's credibility with coworkers can also be jeopardized. When an external consultant is retained without his or her input, the internal consultant has limited choices. The limited choices include the following:

- Making the best of it
- Trying to meet with the external consultant to talk about the scope of work and set the parameters for the working relationship between the internal and external consultant
- Making another pitch to the person hiring the external consultant in an effort to influence the choice of the external consultant, or at least to meet the final candidates; this is a good time to reiterate how a truly collaborative effort can benefit the employer
- Enlisting the help of the internal consultant's patron or advocate to influence the choice of an external consultant

In rare instances, the internal consultant may be tempted to quit or to sabotage the efforts of the external consultant. Such "get even" tactics are likely to do the most damage to the internal consultant. Before undertaking any such scheme, talk the situation through with a trusted mentor, colleague, or friend. Seek another outlet for whatever anger or frustration may arise.

Likewise, the external consultant should approach with care an assignment involving internal consultants. Clarification of the work to be undertaken and delineation of responsibilities for the internal and external consultant must be insisted on by the external consultant. The external nurse consultant must be assured of "good chemistry" with the internal nurse consultant and that the internal consultant has the skills and expertise to do the job and the support of management in bringing another consultant to the assignment. The external consultant will want to ensure that the assignment is truly a collaborative one and not one in which the external consultant is brought in to support a weak internal consultant.

Should the Internal Consultant Build an External Practice?

The internal nurse consultant will very likely be tempted to branch out and test the external consulting waters. In fact, it might be enticing to try to consult outside on a part-time basis while maintaining employment status and an internal consulting role. Having a "foot in both camps" gives the nurse consultant the security of employment on the one hand and an opportunity to try a more independent role on the other.

A chance to consult outside of the employing organization might arise at the behest of a former patient, a vendor, or a colleague. An external role might be urged on the internal consultant by a manager or administrator who wants to lend the nurse's skills and expertise to a satellite facility or an independent company as a gesture of good will or as a service to the community. However the external consulting work comes about, there are several things to keep in mind:

- Be sure the employer is aware of the external consulting work.
- Consult employment policies to be sure that "moonlighting" is not prohibited.
- Do not do external work on internal time, or use internal resources to support external activities.
- Keep careful records of payments received and expenses incurred for external work.
- Ensure that professional liability insurance covers external work.

The Employer.   Employees often do not want to tell employers about external work activities, believing it is none of the employer's business how hours away from the employment site are spent. Employers may have a clear policy prohibiting "moonlighting," although there is debate about the legality of such a prohibition. There can be anxiety on the employer's part about the internal consultant's loyalty to the employing organization. The authors urge the internal nurse consultant to share the intent to consult externally so that objections or misconceptions about the work can be dealt with at the outset. In addition, any appearance of having secrets or sneaking around can be avoided, and fears that the employer's time or resources will be used for external work can be dispelled.

Should the internal nurse consultant want to test the external consulting marketplace, she or he may want to stipulate to the employer that the external work will consume a set number of hours per week; that no consulting will be done for competitors; and that none of the employer's resources will be used for the external work unless there is a special situation (e.g., the employer has asked the internal nurse consultant to take on an external project as a community service).

Record Keeping.   The internal nurse consultant who develops an external consulting practice should keep meticulous records of revenue earned and expenses incurred for external consulting work. Such records have a threefold purpose. First, the internal nurse consultant will have to pay taxes on money earned outside the employment setting. A careful record of expenses, such as mileage, supplies, and postage, will prove helpful in calculating business deductions when completing tax returns. Second, records of income and expenses can be enlightening to the internal consultant in determining how much an external business venture can cost. Third, the internal consultant will get a sense of the demand for the skills and expertise she or he wishes to offer in the external marketplace.

Professional Liability Insurance.   Every nurse consultant, whether self-employed or employed by an agency or institution, should have professional liability insurance. Anyone can be sued for malpractice. Patients are often willing to sue over undesirable treatment or care outcomes, and clients may be tempted to sue over defective advice. Given the litigious nature of today's society, all nurse consultants should consider malpractice insurance a good investment in making the future secure and providing peace of mind in the present.

The internal nurse consultant may have professional liability insurance as an employee benefit. The internal consultant should inquire what kind of coverage the employer provides. Often there are gaps in an employer's policy. For example, attorneys' fees and court costs may not be covered by an employer's policy, or there may not be adequate coverage. Blanket settlement limits might be spread among all employees. Cost-cutting efforts in health care institutions may also have resulted in decreased coverage. For all of these reasons, the nurse consultant needs to carry professional liability insurance or a policy that supplements the employer's policy.

Most coverage provided by employers does not protect the nurse outside the employer's workplace. Thus, the internal nurse consultant providing services outside the employment setting is wise to secure personal liability protection. Some professional liability policies cover the small-business owner (e.g., the nurse consultant). The coverage often includes legal fees; court costs; loss of earnings for court appearances; and general liability for claims occurring on business property, for auto accidents, and so forth. Careful scrutiny of the employer's policies and then the careful purchase of supplemental coverage is a must for the internal nurse consultant.

SUMMARY

The internal nurse consultant is an employee who provides advice and counsel in the work setting. The internal consultant can be a rich resource across facilities or units within a facility helping with education or patient care. The internal nurse consultant might be an intrapreneur, always experimenting and creating new ways of work.

The skill set for the internal consultant closely matches that of the external consultant: good listening, communication, and problem-solving skills. Many of the processes used by the external consultant are similar to those used by the internal consultant: clarity about projects to be undertaken, affirmation of the parameters of the work in writing, a communications link with those who are responsible for the consulting work undertaken, and adherence to time lines.

Difficulties encountered by the internal consultant can include perceptions of bias or being perceived as part of the problem. On the other hand, the advantages of internal consulting include a steady paycheck, an accessible network of peers and colleagues, and support services. Like the external consultant, the internal consultant must be vigilant for consulting opportunities and may have to prove his or her abilities repeatedly.

Although the role of the internal consultant is a fairly new one, an internal consulting practice can be a fresh approach to institutional nursing practice, helping the nurse remain enthusiastic about his or her work and providing new avenues for application of knowledge and skills. The internal nurse consultant can bring additional value to the employer through sharing expertise, knowledge, or talent beyond the assigned area of work. A consulting practice within the employment setting can serve as a testing ground for acquiring and honing consulting skills that might be later used in an entrepreneurial venture. In an era in which employing organizations are rapidly changing and employment opportunities are constantly shifting, building an internal consulting practice may be one way to thrive and survive in the days ahead.

REFERENCES

Block, P. (1981). *Flawless consulting*. San Diego: Pfeiffer & Co.

Champy, J. (1995). *Reengineering management*. New York: Harper Collins.

Lange, F. C. (1987). *The nurse as an individual, group or community consultant*. Norwalk, CT: Appleton-Century-Crofts.

Orsburn, J., Moran, L., Musselwhite, E., & Zenger, J. (1990). *Self-directed work teams: The new American challenge*. New York: Irwin.

Pinchot, G. (1985). *Intrapreneuring*. New York: Harper & Row.

Manion, J. (1990). *Change from within: Nurse intrapreneurs as health care innovators*. Kansas City: American Nurses Association.

Manion, J. (1994). How to innovate from within. *American Journal of Nursing, 94*, 1.

5

Starting a Consulting Business

Starting a consulting business is an exciting venture. Becoming an entrepreneur means being among those who "plan, organize, finance, and operate their own businesses" (Church, 1984, p. 1). This initial excitement can wear off, however, in the face of the myriad of decisions that need to be made and implemented.

Among the decisions that must be made by the new entrepreneur are what to name the business, how to organize it, how to finance it, and how to operate it. These and other aspects of starting a business are the focus of this chapter.

NAMING THE BUSINESS

The first decision generally facing the new entrepreneur is what to name the business. The business name reflects the individual or individuals involved in it and must wear well over the years. The business name must fit the nurse consultant and the type of consulting he or she does.

Many nurse consultants name their businesses after themselves. There are several advantages to that approach. Unlike a product, consultation is a service, and generally a service performed by an individual whose name is known to the client. The "product" in consultation is the relationship between client and consultant, and the nurse consultant's name personalizes that relationship.

It is much more difficult to choose a name other than the nurse consultant's and then market that impersonal name to potential clients so that they will associate it with the nurse consultant. If an impersonal company name is chosen, for example "Nursing Consultation Services," then a search for other companies with that name must be conducted to ascertain whether the name has been registered previously. The secretary of state's office at the state level and the Patent and Trademark Office at the federal level should be contacted to initiate this search.

Many nurse consultants choose names, such as "Smith and Associates," that embody their own names and at the same time allow for potentially adding others to the firm. Others choose only their own names: "Ruth Marshall, Nurse Consultant." In the case where more than one individual is involved in the business, the name might be "Henry and Jones, Inc." or "Henry and Jones Nurse Consultants." It also is possible to combine an individual's name with an impersonal company name, such as "Henry and Jones Pediatric Nursing Consultation Services." An impersonal company name, however, might be appropriate when the company has more than one or two nurse consultants.

Once the name has been decided on, it should be used in everything related to the business (e.g., letterhead, business cards, and business checks). Concomitantly, everything related to the business should be kept separate from the consultant's personal affairs.

FINANCING THE BUSINESS

Most nurse consultants do not start their business on a sound financial footing—it may be years before that happens. In the meantime, some funds are needed to allow the nurse consultant to conduct business. Some nurse consultants are fortunate enough to have personal reserves that will allow them to underwrite the business, and some may have friends and relatives who are willing to invest in the start-up business. Another way of generating funds to launch a business is to consult part-time while still employed and on the employer's payroll, perhaps as an internal nurse consultant or intrapreneur (see chapter 4). During this period of part-time consultation, the nurse consultant would carefully place all money received for those activities in a reserve fund to be used when the business is initiated full-time.

Should those funding avenues not be feasible, other funding sources are available; including commercial banks, finance companies, the government, venture capitalists, and others (Bangs, 1982). Each of these sources offers advantages and disadvantages, as described below.

Commercial Banks

Commercial banks lend money to new businesses, although not without some difficulty. Loans for small businesses, particularly new and untested ones, are notoriously hard to obtain (Kamoroff, 1987).

Most bankers prefer to initiate financial arrangements with those who are already their customers, particularly customers with whom they have enjoyed a pleasant relationship in the past. Thus the nurse consultant would first approach a bank where he or she has a personal account, such as checking, savings, mortgage loan, or certificates of deposit. Bankers will make decisions about lending money on the strength of an entrepreneur's business plan (see the section on business plans later in this chapter).

The advantage of obtaining funds from a bank is that the nurse consultant is not obligated to friends and family; nor will the bank as investor seek part ownership of the business, as might be the case with a relative or friend who is investing in the business. Interest rates for commercial loans are higher than those for personal loans, so the nurse consultant may wish to apply for a personal loan, using personal property as collateral.

One example of the latter approach that has gained in popularity recently is the home equity loan, in which the individual's home is pledged as collateral for a loan against its value. A major disadvantage of this approach is that the individual's house is in jeopardy if he or she defaults on the loan.

Finance Companies

Finance companies generally are less difficult than banks to deal with when seeking funds. The downside, however, is that finance companies charge substantially higher interest rates than banks (Tuller, 1992). Also, most loans are short term, so that someone seeking money from a finance company should have predetermined that the funds will be used only for a short time and repaid as quickly as possible.

Government

The federal government has loan programs, grant programs, and loan guarantee programs for businesses. One of the best known of these is the Small Business Administration (SBA), which offers loan guarantees with commercial banks and other assistance. Individuals must meet stringent requirements, and there is a great deal of paperwork, but in some instances working with the SBA may be the individual's only source of funding for a business.

The SBA also offers free counseling through the Service Core of Retired Executives (SCORE). This group consists of retired individuals who possess expertise in many areas of business and work with entrepreneurs on a one-to-one basis. Often, the SBA and SCORE will offer workshops on starting a business that cover topics such as business structure, insurance, business plans, and accounting. Specific information about current SBA programs can be obtained by contacting the SBA.

State and local governments also offer programs to assist budding entrepreneurs. A local chamber of commerce or college or university small business development center can provide this information.

Venture Capitalists

Venture capitalists are individuals who invest in small businesses, particularly those that are expected to grow rapidly and offer a good return on the investment. The key to attracting venture capitalists lies in the business plan, which shows the potential for growth and attractive financial returns. The disadvantage of accepting funds from this source is that the venture capitalist almost always wants to be a part owner of the company in which he or she is investing.

Other Sources of Financing

Other ways to raise needed start-up funds include borrowing on insurance policies, using cash advances from credit cards, cashing in certificates of deposit, redeeming bonds, selling stock, and so on. These ways will provide ready cash but also carry risks. The savvy entrepreneur does not view these risks lightly, for the business as well as personal assets can be jeopardized if the business venture fails.

The amount of money needed to start a consulting business varies. Money may be needed only to print letterhead stationery and business cards if the nurse consultant already owns business equipment, such as a computer, printer, facsimile, and a telephone answering machine.

Efforts should be made to keep initial outlays to a minimum. Additional supplies and equipment can be purchased once money starts to come in from clients. Whenever possible, money should be allocated to a reserve fund to ensure that the nurse consultant is able to meet living expenses in periods where business income is minimal. Conventional wisdom indicates that it may be between 3 to 5 years before a business begins to show a profit, so it is essential to have a well-thought-out plan to ensure sufficient revenue to meet living and other expenses during that period.

CHOOSING THE BUSINESS STRUCTURE

One of the important decisions that must be made by the nurse consultant going into business is the structure of the business. The structure under which the business is established has both legal and tax implications. Professional as well as personal concerns also influence the choice of business structure. Following is a discussion of the types of business structure and the advantages and disadvantages of each.

Sole Proprietorship

A sole proprietorship is the simplest and easiest business structure to set up and maintain. In a sole proprietorship, one individual is the company. This means that for legal and tax purposes, there is no distinction between the nurse consultant and the business, even though there are separate records for personal accounts and business accounts. A sole proprietor does not experience any of the difficulties—or expenses—involved in incorporating the business, filing reports with government agencies, and so on. However, the sole proprietor does not have the protection offered by incorporation. Any business liabilities are transferred directly to the individual. Another disadvantage of a sole proprietorship is that potential clients may not perceive the company as established.

Tax obligations for the sole proprietor are managed by filing Schedule C with the individual's Internal Revenue Service (IRS) Form 1040. Losses from the consulting firm thus can be used to offset other expenses.

Recently, the IRS has begun scrutinizing Schedule C returns more closely; business losses reported for 3 to 5 years may trigger an audit. Many businesses require at least 3 to 5 years before they are profitable, and consultation businesses are no exception. Thus it is important for the nurse consultant to remain apprised of IRS "red flags" and be prepared to address them if necessary.

Documentation is critical in this structure, as in other forms of business. Careful records will allow the nurse consultant to track income and expenses accurately and will be of immeasurable value in case of an IRS audit.

Partnership

In a partnership, two or more individuals join together to do business. Partners may or may not choose to incorporate a business. Partners should have complementary skills—if one is expert in marketing, for example, the other might focus on administration. It is essential for partners to draw up an agreement that covers what each will contribute (e.g., time, talent, and money) to the business, how profits and losses will be shared, and what will happen to the business if one partner wants out or is incapable of continuing in the business because of disease, disability, or death.

The partners' share of profits from the business is taxable to the individuals involved. The business profits are reported to the IRS on Schedule K-1 (IRS Form 1065). The IRS uses these forms to compare business earnings with profit reported on the partners' tax returns. Any discrepancies will result in action—ranging from a reminder letter to an audit.

Corporation

C Corporation.   Several types of corporations exist. One type is the C corporation, which is a separate, legal entity with officers, a board of directors, stockholders (who may be officers or directors as well), and bylaws.

Articles of incorporation must be filed with the secretary of state in the state in which the corporation is doing business. A filing fee also must be paid. Often, an attorney is engaged to file these articles of incorporation, adding to the cost of the process. It is possible for the owners of the corporation to file their own articles of incorporation; the necessary forms and instructions are available from the secretary of state's office.

Individuals who are stockholders in a corporation are protected from liability; officers, however, are not protected. Officers may be sued by stockholders for unfair practices or fined by the government for a variety of infractions.

Corporations typically are inundated with the paperwork necessary to maintain a separate entity: writing bylaws, holding annual meetings of stockholders, and filing taxes and annual reports with the state. Corporations, however, have the advantage of being able to sell stock to raise capital. Corporations also can grow into an asset for the owners when the business is sold.

The tax liability for a corporation is paid directly by the corporation, although any dividends paid to the stockholders are reported on the individual's tax return and taxed at the individual's tax rate.

Subchapter S Corporation.   The subchapter S corporation (*S-corp.*) is a variation of a C corporation and often is the preferred form for a start-up consulting firm. A business must meet the following 4 criteria to qualify as an S-corp.:

1. It must be organized in the United States.
2. It must offer only one class of stock.
3. It must not have more than 35 shareholders.
4. Its shareholders must be individuals and citizens of the United States.

Individuals involved in an S-corp. have the protection from liability of a corporation, but the S-corp. is not taxed as is a corporation. Instead, as in a partnership, profits and losses from the S-corp. are passed through to the shareholders and are reported on their individual tax returns. The tax form used by individuals involved in an S-corp. to report their profits or losses is Schedule E. The S-corp. also reports its income and expenses to the IRS on Form 1120.

Unlike sole proprietorships and partnerships, the two forms of corporations have an unlimited lifetime; that is, they do not depend on the lifetimes of the principals involved. This allows the corporations more flexibility in relationships with other corporations, such as joint ventures, mergers, and acquisitions.

PAYING BUSINESS TAXES

Paying taxes is a necessary part of doing business as an entrepreneur. The tax burden may be lessened, however, by doing business as a sole proprietor or S-corp. and by not having employees. Regardless of the form of business selected by the nurse consultant, any employees who are paid wages or salaries also are subject to withholding of state and federal taxes, social security Federal Insurance Contributions Act (FICA) taxes, Medicare, and unemployment taxes. These taxes also apply when the nurse consultant is an employee, whether self-employed (as in a sole proprietorship or partnership) or employed by the corporation.

Nurse consultants practicing as sole proprietors, partners, or owners of an S-corp. are required to pay estimated taxes if all their sources of income and self-employment tax will exceed taxes paid through withholding and credits by $500 or more. These estimated federal taxes are paid in quarterly installments on April, June, September, and January 15. Corporations also pay estimated tax according to a schedule established by the IRS. The due dates for payment of estimated state taxes vary by state.

Estimated taxes and other business taxes are predicated on the calendar year. Therefore, most consultants choose the calendar year (January–December) as their taxable year. Another period can be chosen instead. A fiscal year, which is a "twelve month period ending on the last day of any month other than December" (Kamoroff, 1987, p. 86), also can be used. Tax payment due dates are affected by the taxable year.

The nurse consultant must be certain to adhere to requirements for tax payments. Underpayment of taxes can result in penalties and interest. If income from consultation activities varies over the year, it is wise to seek assistance from an accountant.

KEEPING RECORDS

Keeping accurate and complete records is absolutely essential in a business. Tax return files should be kept indefinitely. Records substantiating those tax returns (W-2 forms; 1099s) should be kept for 7 years.

Records pertaining to property owned by a business (an office building) should be kept indefinitely. Written records also should be kept for improvements to the property. Property appraisals and tax depreciation schedules are included in these records, to be kept indefinitely.

These guidelines for keeping records apply whether the records are kept by hand or on a computer. The nurse consultant should confer with his or her accountant or tax adviser for additional assistance related to what types of business records must be kept and how long they must be kept.

CONVEYING AN IMAGE

The image a business projects is as important as the name of the business and its structure. The image of the business conveys its personality and core values. The nurse consultant must initially identify the image he or she wishes to business to convey and then work to reinforce that image in everything related to the business, from how the firm's services are marketed to how mistakes are handled. To build an image for a consulting business, the nurse consultant must (Brown, 1994, p. 207):

1. Know what attributes are most important to potential clients
2. Decide which of these attributes are characteristic of the nurse consultant
3. Know what sets the nurse consultant's services apart from those of competitors

The business's image is conveyed to current and potential clients and other audiences through promotional material, letterhead stationery, and business cards. It is important that all print materials portray a professional look because they often establish the first impression of the nurse consultant and sometimes may be the potential client's only point of contact.

Letterhead stationery can be inexpensively printed at a quick-print shop, but some thought should go into its design. Information on the letterhead should include the business name, address, telephone and fax numbers, and an e-mail address, if one is available. The consultant's name should also be included, if it is not apparent from the company name. The nurse consultant may also wish to add some information on his or her specialty area of practice, but care should be taken not to use a "laundry list."

This letterhead information should be printed in a type size no smaller than 12 points in an easily readable font, such as Helvetica or Times Roman. Save the fancy typefaces and boldface or italics for purposes other than conveying a business image. Also, using graphics on the letterhead, other than the business logo, if one is available.

The ink should be dark (e.g., blue or black). The letterhead paper should be white or a neutral color, such as a variation of cream or gray. A contrasting color ink can add to the look of the letterhead, but showiness or extravagance does not garner clients (Tuller, 1992); indeed, a perceived excess may deter clients. Envelopes of the same paper as the letterhead should be printed as well.

Business cards should be designed to complement the letterhead, but the cards should be printed on heavier stock than the letterhead.

Printing costs are reduced when printing in quantity, but an initial order should purposely be small. If any information changes, the entire order will have to be redone, so purchasing small quantities works best. It may be tempting to print letterhead and business cards on a laser printer as needed, but although these are convenient and inexpensive, they are no substitute for letterhead professionally printed on a commercial press.

DECIDING WHERE TO WORK

The nurse consultant must decide where to work. Most individuals begin by working at home simply for convenience, but there are many factors to consider when deciding where to locate a consulting practice.

Working at Home

Working at home is convenient, but it may not be the best place to meet with clients. The lack of distinction between personal and professional lives also may make focusing on work difficult: There always are dishes to be washed and floors to be vacuumed, and the nurse consultant who locates the office in the corner of the master bedroom will surely experience these distractions.

Ideally, a separate room will be established for the office, and if that room has a separate entrance, so much the better. If not, however, the office still can be arranged to separate it clearly from the living quarters. If a room can be entirely devoted to an office, it will be easier to distinguish between personal and professional activities. If the office must be in a room devoted to other purposes, choose a room that is used for those purposes as little as possible—a guest room, for instance, rather than a family member's bedroom.

Locating an office in a home has tax benefits as well. Current IRS regulations allow for deductions for the space in a home used for business purposes, but the consultant should be aware that the IRS closely scrutinizes this deduction, and it can trigger an audit. The space must be used exclusively on a regular basis for business purposes. Home office space is deductible only if it is the place where most of the consultant's work is conducted; therefore, a nurse consultant who works primarily in the client's location (e.g., hospital or long-term care facility) cannot deduct the costs of the home office.

The tax deduction for home office space is calculated by adding all direct costs for operating and maintaining the home office. These direct costs include, but are not limited to, utilities, repairs, and insurance. In addition, a share of general home expenses can be deducted. The share is based on the percentage of the home's total area that is used for business purposes. For example, if the home is 2,250 square feet and the bedroom used for an office is 225 square feet, 10% of general home expenses can be deducted. General home expenses include but are not limited to cleaning, real estate taxes, repairs, and depreciation.

A word of caution, however: Although depreciating the part of the home used for business reduces tax liability, it also lowers the cost basis of the house. When the house is sold, capital gain is calculated on net sales less the depreciated value of the house. Deducting depreciation lowers immediate tax liability but increases capital gain and thus is likely to increase tax liability when the house is sold. It may be wise to consult an accountant or tax expert for advice in deducting depreciation to determine whether the short-term advantage will be outweighed by the potentially negative long-term effects.

At a minimum, a nurse consultant working from home will need the following equipment:

1. Desk and comfortable office chair
2. Computer and printer
3. Fax machine (or a fax-modem in the computer)
4. Telephone with a separate business line
5. Answering machine for the telephone
6. Filing cabinet or other means of storage for office files

The computer equipment should be state-of-the-art. There are many ways to save on office equipment, but purchasing an underpowered computer is not one of them. The key to selecting the right computer is getting educated about computer technology, then defining needs, and then selecting a reputable dealer who will provide service and support following the purchase.

Computer software should also be state-of-the-art. It generally is best to purchase brand name software packages that have been on the market for years and offer telephone support and automatic upgrades. Obscure software may do the job as well as better-known software, but there may not be someone in the immediate vicinity who can solve problems that arise.

The nurse consultant probably will want a word-processing program for letters, proposals, and reports. A bookkeeping program will allow tracking of income and expenses and managing the business checkbook. A spreadsheet program will permit financial forecasting, and a graphics program will allow the nurse consultant to prepare slides and transparencies for presentations.

The telephone system should allow reception of voice and fax transmissions. Equipment is available that distinguishes between a voice call and a fax call. This allows the use of one telephone line for both voice and fax transmissions, thus eliminating the need for a separate telephone line for the fax machine. The nurse consultant also must be able to receive calls when away from the office; thus a telephone answering machine is essential. Program the answering machine with a businesslike message; encourage callers to leave a message. If possible, the nurse consultant should update the message daily, giving a time when he or she will be available to call back or to receive a call if the caller does not wish to leave a message.

Many individuals do not like voice mail, preferring instead to talk with an individual directly. If the nurse consultant is aware that his or her potential clients fall into that category, it may be worthwhile to employ an answering service to which calls can be forwarded when the nurse consultant is away from the office.

The technology chosen for the nurse consultant's office should be selected on the basis of financial considerations as well as how it will meet clients' needs. Not all of the office equipment needs to be purchased at once; equipment can be leased with an option to purchase, to reduce the initial outlay, or can be purchased once the amount of revenue warrants that. If current clients do not communicate by fax, there is no need to purchase a fax machine initially. If clients do not need presentations with audiovisuals, then a graphics software program may not be necessary. However, equipment should not be purchased solely on the basis of current clients' needs; future clients should also be considered.

It may be necessary for the nurse consultant to have a photocopying machine, although many stand-alone fax machines can make photocopies as well. In addition, the nurse consultant will need a bookkeeping system and miscellaneous office supplies.

If the consultant's practice is clinical, then other office equipment, such as an examining table, stethoscope, or sphygmomanometer, may be necessary. If the business is educational in nature, then equipment such as an overhead or slide projector may be required.

Renting Office Space

Renting office space is useful in making clear the distinction between personal life and professional life. If the nurse consultant regularly meets with clients in the office rather than in the client's location, renting office space may be the only option for locating the business. Renting office space also gives the nurse consultant the opportunity to choose a location that is convenient for clients or provides maximum visibility to passersby.

Renting office space is more expensive than working at home. The costs for renting or leasing office space are tax deductible, but they also contribute greatly to overhead and thus decrease profits. The terms of a lease for office space may also prevent the nurse consultant from moving elsewhere when he or she needs or wants to move.

In some cities, office space is available that includes services such as photocopying, fax, and secretarial support; this is often described as "executive" office space. The cost is higher than renting "bare" space but may be less than purchasing the services separately.

Working in an office away from home allows the nurse consultant to project a professional image, and, if it is an office with similar professionals, to share ideas and projects. It does contribute greatly to overhead, however, and thus increases the amount of time the nurse consultant must be working at billable rates.

By and large, choosing where to locate an office is a personal decision that should be based on the consultant's knowledge of his or her preferences. Some individuals find they are less productive at home than in a typical office setting; some find the daily commute to work tiresome; some feel comfortable working in blue jeans, whereas others do not; and some find working home alone isolating, whereas others are at their peak when free from the usual office distractions. Locating an office at home for financial reasons is as legitimate as renting office space downtown in order to feel successful and confident.

SELECTING VENDORS AND SUPPLIERS

In business, the nurse consultant will be working with a variety of individuals who will provide products and services. These individuals include an attorney (see chapter 8), accountant, printer, and banker, among others. Selecting these individuals appropriately is critical to the success of the business.

The nurse consultant most likely already has established many of these relationships in his or her past personal and professional dealings. In the event that these individuals are not able to meet the new demands of the business, however, it may be necessary to seek out new relationships.

The best place to start is with individuals already in the consultant's network. Others can refer an accountant or attorney whom they know. Obtaining more than one reference is advisable. The nurse consultant then can interview several potential candidates to determine compatibility of personalities, ascertain fees and areas of expertise, and make a decision.

Suppliers of products, such as office supplies or printing services, are chosen in a similar way. Suppliers can be asked to bid on a job, and the decision is then made on the basis of price or delivery time. Wherever possible, relationships should be established with a view toward the long-term benefits for both parties. In such a mutually beneficial relationship, a supplier may use the nurse consultant as a reference for his or her work, and the nurse consultant can be assured of getting the best service for the money.

DEALING WITH FEES

Setting Fees

Setting appropriate fees for consulting services is an important part of doing business. A fee that is too low means the nurse consultant may not generate sufficient income to support the business. A fee that is too high may price the nurse consultant out of the market. A realistic fee, however, indicates that the client can expect a high-quality service—an acceptable "return on the client's investment."

It is difficult, if not impossible, to determine how much other nurse consultants charge for their services; fees are a well-kept secret. Only if the nurse consultant is contracting for the services of another nurse consultant can he or she discover the other consultant's fees. Only occasionally does a nurse consultant reveal his or her fees. General information about fees can be obtained from the "Directory of Nurse Consultants" published in the *Journal of Nursing Administration* (JONA) on a semiannual basis. Nurse consultants are listed the directory by category, such as "staff development," "quality assurance," "management development," and others. Some of these individuals reveal their consultation fees—in a recent directory, most individuals in the directory stated that the fee was "negotiable."

In the survey of nurse consultants conducted by the authors in mid-1995 and described in detail in chapter 1, respondents indicated a range of hourly fees from less than $100 per hour to between $400 to $500 per hour. Most of the 128 respondents (53, or 41%) charge between $100 and $200 per hour. Some of the respondents did not answer this item, however, pointing up the difficulty of obtaining financial information from consultants about their fees.

Some of these respondents (114, or 89%) also provided their daily fees ranging from less than $500 per day to $3,000 to $3,500 per day. Some of the consultants (27, or 24%) charge fees between $750 to $1,000 per day, although nearly as many (25, or 22%) charge from $500 to $750 per day.

Unfortunately, no item in the survey asked consultants how they calculated these fees. Nor were respondents asked to describe how they decided to increase their fees from time to time.

Once fees are established, it is not wise to negotiate them. If a client can persuade the nurse consultant to lower the price, then the client naturally will think the fee was inflated in the first place and may wonder why the nurse consultant did not simply offer the lower price at the start. Sometimes a client may suggest that a nurse consultant's competitor will do the work for less money. If the nurse consultant is certain that the quoted fee is reasonable and fairly reflects the work to be done, he or she is advised to acknowledge the difference in fees but remain firm. If, however, it is likely that the time required has been overestimated, or there are advantages to be gained by lowering the fee and getting the work, the nurse consultant may choose to reduce the proposed charge for the consultation. Steps should be taken to ensure that there actually is a competitor for the business; the client may be using a fictitious competitor as a ploy to reduce the cost of a project. Experience in negotiation (see chapter 2) and in the field of consultation will aid the nurse consultant in gauging when there is likely to be a bona fide rival for a consultation project.

In general, fees should be established to ensure a fair profit for the nurse consultant's work. As such, the fee must be reasonable and in line with competitors' fees.

Fees that lead the market—that is, fees that are more than consultants usually charge for the same or similar work—may lead to loss of business. Still the nurse consultant should not hesitate to charge a fee that leads the market if he or she has a skill that is scarce in the marketplace, or if his or her skills add considerable value to the consultation assignment.

Fees that lag behind the market are fees below what other consultants charge for the same or similar work. Nurse consultants new to the business or those who consult part-time in addition to regular employment may be tempted to undercut the prices charged by already practicing consultants, to woo business away from others or to get new clients. One serious drawback to this practice is that the nurse consultant will eventually want to charge a competitive fee but then may find it difficult to raise fees, because clients are used to lower rates.

Sometimes the client will have an already established fee in mind for a project. The consultant may wish to ask the client about such a price range. On more than one occasion, the authors have elicited this information or other clues about what the competition has proposed for the project, simply by making an inquiry. Care should be taken, however, not to engage in price-fixing or collude in setting fees—these activities may set the stage for violation of antitrust laws.

According to Shenson (1990), fees are set on the basis of a process that involves four steps:

1. Establishing a rate for daily work, which is the value of the time spent by the consultant and others on the project
2. Determining the expenses of doing business
3. Determining what percentage of the consultant's budget should be devoted to overhead
4. Setting a level of profit.

Establishing a Daily Rate. Establishing a daily rate depends on what the nurse consultant's time is worth. If the nurse consultant decides that his or her time is worth a salary of $50,000 per year, for example, the daily rate is calculated by dividing the annual salary by a realistic number of days the nurse consultant can expect to be paid. A year equals 365 days; deleting weekends (Saturday and Sunday) leaves 260 work days per year. A nurse consultant who plans to be paid for those 260 days each year has a daily rate of $192.31 ($50,000 divided by 260).

Realistically, however, nurse consultants generally are not paid each weekday of the year. So a better daily rate might be calculated for a smaller number of paid days. For example, expecting to be paid 4 of every 5 days per year may provide a more achievable daily rate of $239.44.

Working 4 of every 5 days means the nurse consultant is working almost exclusively for clients, which also may not be very realistic. Some nurse consultants agree that "if you're lucky," you'll consult 10 of every 21 working days in a month, "and then you're working pretty hard" (Brown, 1994, p. 94). Given that average (consulting 10 days a month), the nurse consultant's daily rate then is $416.67; this could be rounded up to $425 or $450, or rounded down to $400.

Determining Expenses: Calculating Overhead. Overhead includes all expenses related to doing business that are fixed costs. Fixed expenses are those that remain at a certain level regardless of whether the nurse consultant is working or not. Expenses such as rent, utilities, payments on leased equipment, payroll, and marketing are examples of fixed costs. Direct expenses, by contrast, vary with the project; these costs include photocopying, travel expenses, telephone charges (other than basic monthly service charges, which are fixed costs), and supplies. Some expenses can be characterized as either fixed or direct. A nurse consultant who travels to secure a contract from a potential client might allocate the travel costs to overhead, whereas travel related to a specific project might be charged directly to the client.

Overhead is best converted to a specific percentage of the daily rate and added to the daily rate when project costs are calculated. All of the fixed costs included in overhead should be used in calculating the percentage to be added to the daily rate, even those that are obtained free or at a discount. A nurse consultant whose spouse handles marketing efforts, for example, should include the costs of those marketing efforts when calculating overhead. A nurse consultant who works from home should nonetheless include the cost of office rental in overhead.

Fixed costs that should be considered in calculating overhead include:

- Space
- Assistance—professional and clerical
- Telephone
- Automobile
- Fringe benefits for nurse consultant and staff, if any
- Marketing
- Professional development

Because the costs of overhead must be figured into the fees charged by the nurse consultant, more detail regarding the specific components of overhead is given below.

Space costs.   Although many nurse consultants work at home, rental of space is clearly part of a business's overhead. Therefore, the nurse consultant should calculate the rental or leasing costs of the space occupied at home. This cost can be estimated by reading classified advertisements describing similar space. Realtors also can provide estimates. Include in the figure for office rent the costs of maintaining the office space as well: cleaning, pest control, and utilities. Also include miscellaneous costs of doing business, such as insurance, license fees, and taxes. Regardless of how the cost is calculated, it should be documented for future reference.

Professional or clerical assistance.   Routine tasks performed by individuals who are employees of the nurse consultant or who are under contract to perform specific services for the nurse consultant should be charged to overhead. Project-specific tasks should be charged to the client. For example, answering the telephone is a routine task, whereas typing a progress report is a project-specific task. A professional who designs a computer program for statistical analysis of data is performing a routine task, whereas the same individual who analyzes a client's data using the computer program is performing a project-specific task.

Telephone.   Both basic and long-distance service charges should be included in calculating telephone costs to allocate to overhead. These charges can be allocated in a variety of ways. For example, the nurse consultant can allocate basic telephone service to overhead and charge each client specifically for long-distance service related to a specific project, or a portion of basic services as well as related long distance service can be charged to clients.

Automobile. Costs for using an automobile in the consulting business also can be charged to overhead. Again, the nurse consultant may choose to allocate part of automotive expenses to overhead and part to clients, if the car is used for project-specific activities.

Whether the car is owned or leased, if it is used for business purposes expenses related to its use should be tracked. Use of an automobile for business purposes must be carefully documented. In the event the nurse consultant uses a car extensively for business purposes, it may be cost-effective for the business to purchase the automobile. Then, all mileage accumulated must be for business purposes. If a personal car is used, a record must be kept of the date, purpose of the trip, beginning and ending odometer reading, and the number of miles driven. The IRS requires this documentation as a basis for using a car for business purposes.

Fringe benefits. Fringe benefits should be included in calculating overhead costs. These benefits may include paid vacation or sick time, insurance coverage, retirement plans, and other costs. The nurse consultant should include the costs of these benefits for himself or herself in calculations. The cost of benefits generally ranges from 21% to 33% of an individual's salary (Shenson, 1990).

Marketing. Marketing the consulting business is an essential part of overhead. Without marketing, the business is not likely to grow (see chapter 7). Unless some portion of marketing costs is allocated to overhead, the nurse consultant will, in effect, not be paid on those days when he or she is not billing clients directly. Marketing costs should account for 20% to 30% of overhead.

Professional development. To attract and retain clients, nurse consultants must remain at the cutting edge of their field. The costs for activities to maintain this professional standing can be allocated to overhead. Include in this category the direct costs (e.g., travel, lodging, and registration fees) for attending continuing education courses or academic courses either for credit or not, and other similar activities to maintain or improve skills, both in consulting and in a practice area. Add in the cost of the time to attend these courses—time when the nurse consultant is not billing clients for services. Purchase of publications, such as books, and the cost of subscriptions to journals should be included, as should the cost of dues to the

TABLE 5.1   Overhead Calculation for a Nurse Consultant
with a Daily Rate of $450, Earning $50,000 per Year.

	Monthly ($)
Office rent	400
Clerical services	1,000
(60% charged to overhead)	
Printing/copies	100
Telephone	150
(voice and fax lines; long distance)	
Automotive	250
Fringe benefits (25%)	1,300
Marketing (30%)	1,035
Professional development	100
(dues and publications)	
Supplies	25
Accounting/legal	100
Taxes	800
Equipment	250
Postage	100
Insurance	175
Miscellaneous	400
Total overhead	5,785

Adapted from Shenson, H. (1990). The contract and fee-setting guide for consultants and professionals. New York: John Wiley and Sons. Reprinted by permission of John Wiley & Sons, Inc.

professional association and any specialty organizations to which the nurse consultant may belong.

Table 5.1 illustrates a sample overhead calculation for a nurse consultant. These overhead costs are then added to the consultant's daily rate when calculating project costs. In the example, the nurse consultant's daily rate is $450, and he or she expects to work 10 days per month. Dividing the total overhead of $5,785 by 10 equals $578.50, which is added to the daily rate for a total daily rate of $1,028.50, or rounded up to $1,200, or down to $1,000.

Calculating a Profit Margin.   In addition to the nurse consultant's daily rate, which is the fee for the nurse consultant's time, and a percentage of overhead, it is wise to charge an amount that will be profit. Profit is the purpose of running a business, and it should accrue to the nurse consultant over and above the rate for labor. The range for profit is between 10% and 20% (Shenson, 1990, p. 12). Once these three amounts are determined, the daily fee can be set.

For example, the nurse consultant's daily rate and overhead costs total $1,028.50. Adding 10% ($102.85) profit increases the daily rate to $1,131.35, or again rounded up to $1,200.

Another formula for establishing a daily consulting rate is offered by Walter M. Pyle, a marketing communications consultant in Boston. Pyle says, "Pick a figure you want to make, divide it by 1,500 hours, add a 'load factor' of 100 percent, which covers indirect costs (secretarial support, rent, heat, light, postage, etc.), and then divide that subtotal by .75, which adds a profit equivalent to 25 percent of the total" (Brown, 1994, p. 94). The figure of 1,500 hours represents 72% of 2,080 hours (which is 260 8-hour work days, or 52 5-day work weeks). The public relations industry considers 72% to be a minimum target for billable hours. Under this formula, 28% of a nurse consultant's time is free for other nonbillable activities, such as marketing, professional development, vacation, sick time, and administration.

Using Pyle's formula, the nurse consultant wishing to make $50,000 per year would divide that amount by 1,500 hours, multiply the result by 2, and divide that amount by .75 for a total hourly rate of $88.88 or a daily rate of $711.04 (assuming an 8-hour day), or rounded up to $750 or down to $700. This formula results in a lower daily rate ($700 or $750 rather than $1,200) because of the difference in projected time spent consulting (1,500 hours per year rather than 960).

A beginning nurse consultant may decide to charge less than the daily fee, perhaps choosing to forgo any profit until better established as an expert in the field. An experienced nurse consultant who is in great demand may choose to charge more than the daily fee he or she has determined. Whatever fee is quoted to the client should be inclusive; that is, the minimum amount of financial data should be disclosed (Cohen, 1985). For a fixed-price contract, quote only the bottom line; for a daily-rate quote, offer only the daily rate, not broken down into its respective components of time, overhead, and profit. (Fixed-price and daily-rate fees are explained later in the chapter.)

Cutting Rates

A nurse consultant at any level of experience may decide to cut his or her rate to obtain a contract that is important to build the business. For example, if the nurse consultant specializes in strategic planning and the potential client is a national health care-related organization, not a local one with whom the nurse consultant has previously conducted strategic planning activities, the nurse consultant may choose to discount the usual rate, figuring that the entrée into the national arena is worth a reduced fee. It is wise to remember, however, not to set fees too low, regardless of the motivation, because expenses must be paid, and they can be overwhelming if not offset by sufficient income (Hand, 1995).

Other variations in daily rate depend on geographic area. Nurse consultants on the East and West Coasts, for example, can be expected to charge more than those in the Midwest and South. Nurse consultants in large metropolitan areas (e.g., New York and Chicago) can be expected to charge more than those in smaller cities (e.g., Toledo, OH and Muncie, IN).

Nurse consultants may also not be able to charge their usual fees when working with government clients. Government agencies often have pre-established rates for nurse consultants. These rates may be below those generally charged by the nurse consultant. In that case, there are a few choices. The nurse consultant can attempt to negotiate a "fixed-fee" contract or subcontract some of the work to lower-paid individuals; or the nurse consultant can decline the contract and seek more lucrative work elsewhere.

However, nurse consultants should beware of charging less for services because a client "cannot afford it." Nurse consultants may feel uncomfortable charging fees that actually cover their services and allow a profit. Cutting fees perpetuates the feeling of unworthiness and the practice of undercharging. Two ways of handling this potential problem include determining what effect accepting the contract will have on the nurse consultant's business. If the net effect is positive in the long run, then it may be acceptable to agree to charge less in order to get the contract. Also, the nurse consultant may decide that a percentage of his or her work will be devoted to "charitable" causes and that accepting the contract at a lower fee will fulfill the commitment to contribute to worthy endeavors. This latter approach will also permit the nurse consultant to decline a contract where the financial or other return is not acceptable. The nurse consultant can simply say that the project will exceed the amount of time he or she has budgeted to contribute to charitable causes.

Arranging for Payment of Fees

Once the consultation fee has been determined, the next step is to decide how to arrange payment of the fee. With a short-term consultation—such as assessing a patient, designing a treatment plan, or educating a local hospital staff about interventions in a single day—payment generally is immediate. With a long-term consultation project, however, such as applying for accreditation of an organization as an approver or provider of continuing education in nursing through the American Nurses Credentialing Center—a project of many months' duration—payment may be made in several installments.

Shenson (1990) has suggested six forms of financial relationships between nurse consultant and client:

1. Fixed-price contract
2. Fixed-fee plus expenses

3. Daily rate
4. Time and materials
5. Cost reimbursement
6. Retainer

Fixed-Price Contract.   In a fixed-price contract, the nurse consultant determines what services will be provided (on the basis of the client's needs) for what price. Those services then are provided to the client for the specified fee. The services generally are specified in the contract, and the nurse consultant is expected to deliver those services within the established time frame and within the established budget. Generally, expenses are included in the contract price quoted to the client.

The advantage of a fixed-price contract is that the client knows exactly what the project will cost, so there are no surprises. The advantage to the nurse consultant is that if the work can be performed in less time than projected, or if expenses can be pared, the profit margin rises—often substantially. Conversely, however, if it takes the nurse consultant longer than estimated to complete the project, or if expenses exceed estimates, the nurse consultant may receive less profit, or even lose money.

In the survey of nurse consultants, respondents strongly (57, or 45% of 128 respondents) indicated that if they find that their costs are running over the projected costs in the contract, they absorb the costs. Only a few (8, or 6%) said they would negotiate a higher fee with the client; even fewer (3, or 2%) said they would negotiate a decrease in the work output. Many (35, or 27%) said they would negotiate both the fee structure and the work output. Several respondents revealed that their action would depend on who was to blame for the problem: "If it is my fault, I will absorb [the costs]; if it is [the client's] fault, I'll negotiate a higher fee structure." Ten respondents (8%) indicated that they had never been in this situation, but unfortunately they did not provide any clues to how they had escaped this common experience.

Fixed-price contracts are common in the consulting industry. The risk to the nurse consultant in this type of contract may be obviated by including a clause in the contract that the price may be renegotiated if the scope or character of the work changes during the period covered by the contract.

There are variations of fixed-price contracts. For example, a contract that is expected to last over a long period may include an annual cost-of-living provision. A contract may also include an incentive payment for completion before the established deadline.

Fixed Fee Plus Expenses.   In this type of contract, the nurse consultant may charge the daily rate as a fixed fee, but bill the client for direct expenses (e.g., travel, postage, and printing). This approach is particularly useful when it is difficult to ascertain direct expenses in advance.

The client has the advantage of knowing the price of the services to be provided in the contract but does not know what expenses will cost—which may be a disadvantage. The consultant has the advantage of receiving his or her daily rate, and, if the work is completed sooner than anticipated, of making a profit in addition. The consultant also is assured of reimbursement for all expenses, so increases in expense items that would have been absorbed by the consultant in a fixed-price contract are paid by the client in this arrangement.

Daily Rate. Because fixed-price contracts are risky, many nurse consultants choose instead to charge the client a daily rate. The nurse consultant estimates the amount of time to be devoted to the project as well as the direct expenses associated with the project. The client accepts these estimates but is responsible for paying charges in excess of the estimates. The nurse consultant must be certain to calculate the estimates accurately; the client will expect to pay no more than the amount estimated and may become disenchanted with the nurse consultant if costs greatly exceed the estimates. The nurse consultant may choose then to absorb the extra cost to avoid upsetting the client. Moreover, if the nurse consultant completes the project in less time than anticipated, the client rather than the nurse consultant benefits.

One way to overcome the disadvantages of daily-rate pricing is to estimate the cost of the project in stages: the first stage involves getting to know the client and the expectations regarding the project; the second stage involves actually completing the project on the basis of a set of assumptions (such as what the nurse consultant will do and what the client will do). The first stage of the project is billed at a daily rate and the second at a fixed price, but with some overage in case the project does not turn out exactly as anticipated. The nurse consultant also can negotiate with the client to bill additional hours if the project does not turn out as planned because of changes in the nature of the project or the expectations of the client.

For example, in a contract in which the nurse consultant was engaged to assess the effectiveness of a statewide coordination mechanism for continuing education in nursing, a fixed-price approach—based on an estimate of the amount of time to be devoted to the project by the nurse consultant—was used. Direct expenses were charged to the client in addition. The agreement contained a proviso that if the client did not produce access to sources of needed information, additional charges would be incurred. Thus, when a data-collection session could not be scheduled as planned because of poor attendance by the principals, another visit by the nurse consultant to the client was necessary, and the consultant's additional time and expenses were paid for by the client.

Time and Materials. In this type of contract, the nurse consultant charges the client for labor costs. The nurse consultant pays expenses, however, and then charges the client for them, rather than having the client pay the expenses directly. The nurse consultant generally adds a handling charge to the invoice for expenses to cover the time spent in paying and tracking expenses.

Variations of this type of contract also exist. Sometimes clerical expenses will be treated as expenses rather than included in the nurse consultant's daily rate.

Cost Reimbursement. In this type of arrangement, the client pays all of the project costs directly. The nurse consultant acts as an agent of the client in performing the agreed-on work. Before beginning the project, both client and nurse consultant must agree on the costs.

Variations also occur with this type of contract: The nurse consultant and client can mutually agree on whether the contract will include a fee as well as costs, whether an incentive will be paid, or whether costs will be shared, as when the nurse consultant can benefit from the project to position himself or herself favorably in similar situations in the future.

Retainer. In a retainer-type agreement, the nurse consultant is available to the client when needed. The nurse consultant must be careful to estimate accurately the amount of time to be allotted to the client; underestimating the time means the nurse consultant will have to devote more time than planned and other projects may suffer; underestimating the time also means that the nurse consultant will not receive income for some of the services he or she provides to the client.

Generally payments to nurse consultants on retainer are made on a monthly basis, with the assumption that during some months the client will require more of the nurse consultant's time than others, but that the workload will average out over the period covered by the contract. The retainer payment plan is advantageous to nurse consultants because it guarantees a monthly income. The nurse consultant has an obligation to meet the client's needs and to avoid taking the client for granted. Because both client and nurse consultant must trust each other for a retainer consultation to work, this type of arrangement is less common than many others.

Retainer payments cover only the nurse consultant's time. Generally, expenses are paid directly by the client, although they can be paid by the nurse consultant and then billed to the client.

The fee structure for consultation services, and the method of payment, must be considered before a proposal can be made to a potential client. Knowing what—and how—to charge a client for consultation services leads to a higher level of satisfaction for both client and nurse consultant.

Collecting Fees

Generally, fees are paid on time, as agreed on by consultant and client. Occasionally, however, fees that are due a nurse consultant are not paid in a timely manner. This is particularly true when the consultation activities involve the government (e.g., Veterans Administration, federal agencies; and the military). Sometimes, a client will pay amounts due at the last minute to offset cash-flow problems.

The first step to defend against late payment is to ensure that invoices are submitted as required (e.g., in triplicate, with the purchase order number prominently displayed, to the correct office). Particularly in a government bureaucracy, incorrect submission of paperwork can delay payment interminably (Holtz, 1983).

The second step in ensuring timely payment is to track accounts receivable. Each time an invoice is sent, a notation should be made on a calendar (in writing or on a computer scheduling program) of the due date for payment. On the day payment is due, generally 30 days from the date the invoice was sent, begin tracing the delayed payment. Call the client and inquire about when payment may be expected. If a telephone call does not result in action within a reasonable time (3 to 5 business days), follow up with a letter or fax. This written message can be followed by a telephone call as well, to inquire whether the written message was received and when payment can be expected.

In the highly unlikely event that these methods do not elicit payment, it will be necessary to escalate the demands for payment. A sharply worded letter to the client's superior may generate some action.

Final steps that may be taken include consulting an attorney, taking the client to small claims court (depending on the amount in question), or hiring a collection agency. These latter means are drastic, are almost certain to affect relations between client and consultant adversely, and so should be employed only when other means have failed. The nurse consultant also may wish to balance the potential negative outcome against the amount of money to be collected; it may be that the decision is that the more drastic course is not worthwhile pursuing. Holtz (1983), however, asserts that "If insisting on being paid with reasonable promptness costs you a client, it is a client not worth having" (p. 213).

OBTAINING BUSINESS LICENSES

Businesses in any state require licensing by the appropriate government agencies. Most businesses must have a "local" license, issued by the county in which the business is located. These licenses are usually not expensive;

the cost ranges from a few to several hundred dollars. The county clerk or some other official at city hall can provide details about local licenses.

Some states require that businesses have a state license. Occupational licenses for registered nurses (RNs) are an example of a state license. Most states have sales tax laws that cover any products (e.g., books and videotape programs) sold by nurse consultants. States require employers to meet laws administered by departments of labor. The blue pages of the telephone directory contain listings of state agencies that might have requirements for a nurse consultant's business, and a local business attorney can provide this information as well.

The federal government also requires licenses for businesses. Initially, a new business is required to obtain a federal Employer Identification Number (EIN) unless the business is structured as a sole proprietorship, in which case the proprietor's social security number is used instead of an EIN. Partnerships and corporations must have an EIN.

To obtain an EIN, Form SS-4 is filed with the IRS. There is no fee for obtaining an EIN, and this identification number then is used for all tax returns filed by the business. The EIN should be included on all invoices sent to clients.

Information about necessary licenses to conduct business in a specific location can be obtained from an accountant, a small-business development center associated with a college or university, or an attorney specializing in business law. Although it is time-consuming and often tedious to track down the information needed to obtain the required business licenses and permits, it is far better to do this before running afoul of the laws in a particular community or state.

BECOMING AN EMPLOYER

When a consulting business grows and the nurse consultant is not able to do all the work that needs to be done, it may be necessary to hire others to help. Because of the plethora of paperwork associated with becoming an employer, it may be wiser to seek alternative ways of obtaining needed assistance. For example, the nurse consultant can subcontract work to others who then perform the work as independent contractors. An independent contractor is defined by the IRS as someone who performs services that are not controlled by the employer (that is, the employer does not control what will be done or how it will be done). In the case of an independent contractor, the employer does not provide the tools or the place to work either.

Extreme caution must be taken in defining the work to be done by independent contractors because these arrangements have recently come under scrutiny by the IRS. The IRS has asserted that if the arrangement between two individuals is in fact an employer-employee relationship by definition, it does not matter what the nurse consultant or anyone else calls the arrangement—outsourcing, using an independent contractor, or sub-contracting. The IRS has a free publication (*Circular E—Employer's Tax Guide*) that defines and describes guidelines for employer-employee relationships.

Individuals who are independent contractors are not covered under an employer's workers' compensation. If an independent contractor is injured while performing work for a nurse consultant, the result could be large medical bills or a lawsuit for the nurse consultant.

Money paid to independent contractors over a year's time must be reported to IRS if the amount exceeds $600 or more. Form 1099-Misc. is used for this purpose. The independent contractor must claim this income on his or her tax return as well.

All employers are required to have a federal EIN. All employees are subject to federal tax withholding; thus each employee must complete a Form W-4 to indicate marital status and number of exemptions claimed. These data determine the amount of federal tax to be withheld from the employee's paycheck.

Employers must also withhold social security tax from employees' paychecks. This tax, commonly known as FICA (for Federal Insurance Contributions Act), varies each year but is always a certain percentage of gross pay up to an annual earnings maximum. Employers must match the employee's contribution.

Employers pay these payroll taxes with Form 941; a booklet of these forms is supplied by IRS. The due date for payment depends on the amount to be paid. Amounts less than $500 can be paid quarterly; amounts more than $500 are paid monthly.

Employers also are liable for Federal Unemployment Tax (FUTA). Only the employer pays this tax; employees are not assessed. Unemployment tax is also levied by the state, and the percentage owed to the federal government varies on the basis of the amount paid to the state. Returns are filed annually on Form 940.

Employers must give each employee a form W-2 annually. This form is used by the employee to file his or her own income taxes and covers the employee's gross wages, federal tax withheld, social security tax withheld, and state and local income tax. The employer uses form W-3 to transmit all of the employees' W-2 statements to the Social Security Administration.

Employees' payroll records must be kept separately from other business records. Payroll records should contain data on the following (Kamoroff, 1987):

- Paycheck date
- Check number

- Payroll period
- Hours worked
- Overtime
- Gross pay
- Federal income tax withheld
- Social security tax withheld
- State and local income tax withheld
- Any other withholding (e.g., insurance coverage)
- Net pay

Because of the complexity of the paperwork caused by having employees, the nurse consultant may seek assistance from an accountant to process the payroll. Some computer software programs also reduce much of the burden of calculating payroll taxes and keeping records. Some businesses also "lease" employees or outsource the payroll.

Most employers must comply with the regulations of the Occupational Safety and Health Administration (OSHA), particularly those related to employees' safety. The Fair Labor Standards Act covers the minimum wage that must be paid to employees. The Americans with Disabilities Act also influences employers. Most of these federal programs affect employers with more than 10 employees, but it is prudent to check the provisions of each to avoid penalties for noncompliance.

Employers with more than three employees must provide workers' compensation insurance to cover injuries on the job. An insurance agent can provide information on workers' compensation plans.

DEVELOPING A BUSINESS PLAN

Understanding Business Plans

To grow, develop, and be successful, a business needs a plan. Financing a start-up business also requires a business plan. Sometimes obtaining a lucrative contract or a key employee depends on a business plan. The focus of a business plan is often on securing capital for a new product, service, or enterprise, such as a consultation practice.

Assistance with developing a business plan is available from a variety of sources, such as the nearest library or bookstore, where references that guarantee a painless, successful business plan can be found. The staff of a small-business development center in a college or university also can provide references, and, perhaps more important, review a draft of a business plan and advise on its completion.

Regardless of the assistance available, it is important for the nurse consultant to write his or her own business plan. No one will know or understand the business better than its owner. There is no one best way to write a business plan, but people who write such plans for someone else often use a "boilerplate," forcing information about every company into the same framework. This standardized presentation may not showcase the nurse consultant's business.

A business plan is useful in allowing the business owner—and others— to take an objective, critical, and unemotional view of a business. The business plan also can be used as an operating tool to manage the business or guide it toward success.

Business plans are particularly useful in three areas of a business:

1. In a start-up venture, to obtain financing
2. When additional financing is needed
3. For new activities within a business

Writing a Business Plan

Key points to consider when writing a business plan are to convey the energy and excitement of the business, stress what makes the business unique, and be as honest about negative aspects of the business as about positive ones. Care should be taken not to disparage others in the field, particularly when describing the competition for the nurse consultant's products or services.

Writing the business plan is time-consuming and may best be scheduled over a period of several weeks. A draft of the plan should be reviewed and revisions made before the final plan is written.

A business plan must contain at a minimum the following (Gumpert, 1990; Vogel & Doleysh, 1994):

- Cover page
- Contents page
- Executive summary
- Description of the company
- Target market
- Product or service
- Marketing strategies
- Finances

Cover Page. The cover page of the business plan should include the name of the company, its business address, its telephone number, and the owner's name. Zip codes should be included with addresses and area codes with telephone numbers. Gumpert (1990) stresses the importance of a cover page—a banker is unlikely to look up a company's telephone number in order to offer financing. Gumpert further advises that the cover page contain a copy number, prominently displayed if the plan is to be widely distributed (for example, to banks for potential financing). That way the copies of the plans can be tracked.

Contents Page. Because most business plans tend to be lengthy, a contents page will allow the reader to focus on areas of interest quickly. The pages of the business plan should be numbered, and this pagination should be reflected on the contents page.

Executive Summary. Again because most business plans are long, an executive summary should be prepared for the reader. The executive summary should stress the most important components of the business plan: the target market, current and future services, and financing needs (Vogel & Doleysh, 1994). Then, the reader can explore sections of interest in depth.

Description of the Company. This section of the business plan should describe the company, including how the business was started, its current status, and projections for the future. The principal owners and operators should be described in this section. Include information such as educational background, experience in the field, accomplishments, and abilities. A résumé or curriculum vitae (see chapter 3) can be included as an appendix in the business plan. A job description should be included if the company has more than one principal.

Target Market. In this section, give information on the company's clients, both current and potential; the competition; and marketing efforts that have been implemented or are contemplated. Evidence to substantiate claims about the potential market must be included in this section or, if extensive, added as an appendix.

Product or Service. This section of the business plan should clearly and specifically identify what the company has to offer clients. In the case of a product, such as a continuing education workshop, the course outline and marketing materials provide evidence of the nature of the product. It is more difficult to describe a service, such as "consultation on evaluation." The description of the service offered should be reviewed by individuals not related to the company for clarity before it is included in the business plan.

Marketing Strategies. Here the nurse consultant will describe how he or she intends to reach the target market and convert it into clients. Samples of promotional materials can be used to illustrate marketing strategies. Plans for marketing activities should be detailed (see chapter 7).

Finances.   In this section, a complete financial picture of the company must be presented. Sources of financing should be described. If the company has been in business for a while, past results as well as future projections should be included. This section is accompanied by "cash flow projections, profit-and-loss statements, and balance sheets" (Gumpert, 1990, p. 20).

The business plan should be produced in an easily readable format, preferably on a laser printer. If the plan is produced with a word-processing program, changes and revisions can be made as necessary following review of drafts or of the final product.

It is essential that the appearance of the business plan reflect as favorably on the nurse consultant as does the content.

SUMMARY

Starting a business is an exciting venture, but one that will be more successful if undertaken by a knowledgeable individual who is aware of—and avoids—the pitfalls of inadequate planning. Various steps must be taken in starting a business: Some of these are the same regardless of the business; others are state- or county-specific requirements.

The savvy entrepreneur investigates how to start a business, incessantly asking questions, seeking information, and verifying data until the decisions that must be made can be made easily. Although it requires a great deal of effort initially, once the business is launched, this good start will make it possible to devote time to "taking care of business" rather than fending off problems.

REFERENCES

Bangs, D. H., Jr. (1982). Business planning guide. In B. R. Riccardi & E. C. Dayani (Eds.), *The nurse entrepreneur* (pp. 103–136). Reston, VA: Reston.

Brown, P. C. (1994). *Jumping the job track: Security, satisfaction, and success as an independent consultant.* New York: Crown.

Church, O. D. (1984). *Small business management and entrepreneurship.* Chicago: Science Research Associates.

Cohen, W. A. (1985). *How to make it big as a consultant* (2nd ed.). New York: AMACOM.

Gumpert, D. G. (1990). *How to really create a successful business plan.* Boston: Inc. Publishing.

Hand, L. E. (1995). *Freelancing made easy.* New York: Doubleday.

Holtz, H. (1983). *How to succeed as an independent consultant.* New York: John Wiley & Sons.

Kamoroff, B. (1987). *Small time operator.* Laytonville, CA: Bell Springs.

Riccardi, B. R., & Dayani, E. C. (1982). *The nurse entrepreneur.* Reston, VA: Reston.

Shenson, H. (1990). *The contract and fee-setting guide for consultants and professionals.* New York: John Wiley & Sons.

Tuller, L. W. (1992). *The independent consultant's Q & A book.* Holbrook, MA: Bob Adams.

Vogel, G., & Doleysh, N. (1994). *Entrepreneuring: A nurse's guide to starting a business* (2nd ed.). New York: National League for Nursing Press.

6

Marketing Consultation Services

In addition to having well-developed professional skills, the nurse consultant must be adept at marketing them. In the study of nurse consultants conducted by the authors in 1995, most individuals who responded to the survey revealed that they most needed help with marketing (72 of 128, or 56%) and getting clients (55 of 128, or 43%) when they began their practice as nurse consultants. Although most respondents indicated that they had formal preparation in consulting (through college degree-credit courses or continuing education courses) and informal preparation (through reading, attending workshops, and listening to audiotapes or viewing videotapes), no item asked about whether this preparation included marketing. Thus, this chapter is devoted to an in-depth exploration of marketing and presents one effective way of getting clients.

DEFINITIONS OF MARKETING

Marketing, according to Echeveste (1982), is "a set of activities necessary and incidental to bringing about exchange relationships in our economic system" (p. 44). Kelly (1987), in describing how to market educational programs, refers to Kotler's classic definition of marketing as "the analysis, planning, implementation, and control of carefully formulated programs designed to bring about voluntary exchanges of values with target markets for the purpose of achieving organizational objectives" (pp. 187–188). Drucker (1993) defined marketing as a business purpose or action that creates a customer. According to Ethier (1988), marketing involves "identifying product and service needs and meeting them in a manner consistent with the organization's goals" (p. 107).

Further, Holtz (1992) describes marketing a consultant's services as "hard work" but notes that hard work is generally the secret to success. Alward and Camuñas (1991) note that marketing is "necessary whenever there is a highly competitive, resource-constrained environment" (p. 3), and this description certainly fits nursing and health care today.

MARKETING PLAN

Certainly, the nurse consultant's services will not be in demand unless others (clients) know what those services are and how they may access them. Getting the word out may be hard work for a variety of reasons, not the least of which is that nurses are not used to selling themselves or their services. The consultant will not be successful, however, if others do not contract for his or her services. Thus, it is important for the nurse consultant to develop and implement a marketing plan. Basically, the marketing plan consists of four elements:

1. Services to be offered
2. Clients for those services
3. How the clients can be reached
4. Specific offer to be made (Holtz, 1983).

Determining Services to Be Offered

The services to be offered by the nurse consultant have already been described (see chapter 3). The nurse consultant determines the professional skills and abilities that can benefit the potential client, then pursues a course of action, educationally and experientially, to maintain and continuously improve those skills. In this way, at all times, the client is receiving the best possible, most up-to-date services from the nurse consultant.

Assessing the Potential Clientele

A critical step in ensuring the success of consulting ventures is to decide who are the clients who will avail themselves of the nurse consultant's services. Definition of the potential population to whom marketing efforts will be targeted often is the point at which consulting fails. Holtz (1983) asserts that "Many business failures are traceable to thoughtless and irresponsible sales efforts, made without considering who were the proper prospects for whatever the entrepreneur wished to offer" (p. 76). Indeed, a nurse consultant who does not take seriously the admonition to assess the potential clientele may devote much time, energy, and money on marketing—to the wrong audience—with no results.

Once a target client has been identified, the nurse consultant learns as much as possible about this client. This study of the client population takes the form of assessing the client's actual need for services, how those services might be provided, how likely it is that the client will seek consulting services, what advertising the client is likely to respond to, how receptive the client is to consulting services, and so on. The more the nurse consultant knows about the potential client, the more likely it becomes that the consulting services can be designed for specific needs and that the potential client will take advantage of the services offered.

In a hospital, for example, the clinical nurse specialist as internal nurse consultant or intrepreneur (see chapter 4) may note increased stress on the part of head nurses as a result of lack of adequate staffing: Head nurses are trying to maintain nursing coverage for their units on a daily basis, but the institution is unable to hire sufficient nurses to meet the demand, because of a decline in the number of nurses seeking employment. As a result of this and other characteristics of the work environment, stress is increased and morale severely affected.

The clinical nurse specialist (CNS) knows that one market for stress management services is this group of beleaguered head nurses. The CNS knows, too, that the head nurses have a limited amount of time to devote to stress reduction; they are likely to want a quick fix, but they are highly motivated as a result of their acute discomfort. As a result of knowing the target population, the clinical nurse specialist can plan and implement a 2-hour session on "relaxation techniques," all of which can be used at work. Once their immediate needs have been addressed, the head nurses may be more amenable to devoting efforts to long-range solutions. Had the clinical nurse specialist designed a daylong workshop on "making changes," for example, the results would not have been as positive, because the head nurses had neither the time nor the inclination to assume a project of that magnitude.

In a situation in which the nurse consultant has been approached by an industry to design a teaching program, the consultant would begin by learning about the company, its products, its market, the role of education, the target audience for the proposed program, the resources available, and so on. Such advance knowledge about the company ensures that the nurse consultant will prepare a proposal to meet the company's need for the educational program rather than making unrealistic or inappropriate suggestions.

Although knowing the potential clientele will help the nurse consultant effectively aim toward the right group, the target market may change over time. From offering stress management services to head nurses, for example, the CNS may decide to offer those services to other departments in the hospital, and then to other hospitals and health care agencies in the community. It is equally important to assess when the target group has changed as it is to decide who the client is in the first place, to avoid losing consulting opportunities.

The nurse consultant must devote some time to continuous, ongoing assessment of the target audience for his or her services. Keeping up requires reading the industry literature; talking with individuals in the field; and attending educational, business, and social events in the target industry; and perhaps even in related industries. One successful strategy is to target two to three individuals from the consultant's network to telephone each month and generally discuss what is going on in the industry. Different individuals would be called each month. The average call lasts 5 to 10 minutes and reaps an amazing amount of information and helps the nurse consultant keep in touch with contacts.

Reaching the Clients

Once the target audience has been defined, the next step is to decide how to sell this audience on the nurse consultant's services. This, too, is a critical step. Despite all the good work that went into assessment of specific services to offer and whom to offer them to, if the right market is not reached with the right product, there will be no sale.

The nurse consultant uses knowledge of the target clients to design the appropriate strategies to sell them consulting services. In the hospital setting, the clinical nurse specialist initially may use a "try it—you'll like it" approach, suggesting a quick, guaranteed relaxation technique to a harried head nurse (e.g., "When I'm this stressed, it usually works for me if I take a deep breath, then visualize myself accomplishing an activity that is pending. I see myself being successful in completing the activity and feeling good about what I've done"). The head nurse then tries what was suggested while the clinical nurse specialist observes. On completion of the exercise, the head nurse says, "That helped—thanks!"

It is fairly certain that the head nurse will tell colleagues, who will then approach the clinical nurse specialist for help too. The word spreads, and the target audience now is receptive to more formalized approaches. Word-of-mouth techniques are the most effective advertising, and often they are the most appropriate in a situation as well. In a hospital setting, for example, it would be improbable that the clinical nurse specialist could market stress management services through a brochure or other printed matter.

Initially, the nurse consultant will obtain clients from his or her network of friends, acquaintances, and colleagues. Networking with others to sell services is a difficult form of marketing, but that should not deter the nurse consultant from proceeding with it. Once a comfortable client base has been established, marketing efforts become easier.

These initial marketing efforts are easier if the nurse consultant has had some experience with consulting—while already employed at a health care facility as an internal nurse consultant or intrepreneur (see chapter 4), for example, or if the nurse consultant has a mentor, or one established client or contract. The nurse consultant who has joined with an established consultant can learn marketing strategies from the experienced consultant. Working with an established consultant can result in being able to observe and learn many aspects of the consulting business, not the least of which is marketing. The nurse consultant with specialized expertise or a reputation in the profession also may find initial marketing less difficult than the novice nurse consultant. The nurse consultant with well-established networks can mine them for referrals for business opportunities.

The point must be made here, however, that the nurse may already be providing consultation services of which he or she is unaware. The nurse who provides advice to nursing colleagues on a patient's problem or condition in a hospital is consulting with those colleagues. The staff development educator who plans and implements an educational activity in response to an organizational need is a consultant. The nurse who develops a teaching program on foot care for patients with diabetes and then teaches others to implement the program is, in fact, a consultant.

It may be that the nurse desiring to become a consultant needs to begin the process by viewing his or her activities with an eye toward identifying them as consultation regardless of whether they have been perceived as consultation activities previously. Any instance in which the nurse makes an exchange with another for the purpose of achieving a goal or objective is consultation, and nurses perform numerous consultation activities in their daily work.

Selecting the Specific Offer

Once strategies for reaching the potential clientele have been devised, the nurse consultant next has to decide what specific services will be offered. The nurse consultant's repertoire will contain more areas of expertise than are applicable in any situation, so what is to be offered must be carefully delineated to meet the client's needs most effectively. Again, the nurse consultant uses prior knowledge of the existing needs and the client to achieve this match between his or her skills and what the client wants.

It is tempting to select only one area of expertise on which to focus, but to be successful, the nurse consultant must always be on the "cutting edge," ready to move into other areas when the climate is right. For example, several years ago a plethora of workshops and conferences for nurses appeared on the topic "Death and Dying," spurred primarily by the work of Elisabeth Kübler-Ross. Now, however, although people are still dying and nurses need to deal with this phenomenon in their practice, educational events on that topic are rare. The individual who targeted teaching death and dying as a single area of expertise would soon have found himself or herself with little or nothing to do.

FINDING CLIENTS

The next step after developing a marketing plan is actually finding clients. The nurse consultant's clients are readily defined as individuals, groups, and organizations in need of the specific services that the nurse consultant offers. Finding those clients, however, is an entirely different problem. It is important for the nurse consultant to have a clear idea of the services he or she can offer. This involves identifying specifically what are the nurse consultant's areas of expertise, who is likely to need that expertise, who else could provide that expertise to clients (the nurse consultant's competitors), and why the nurse consultant is a better choice for clients than his or her competitors.

Once this background information is gathered, the nurse consultant is ready to target potential clients. As mentioned earlier, initial clients probably will be those already in the nurse consultant's networks, and they will be easy to contact. (This is also discussed at the end of the chapter.) Other potential clients, however, may not be known to the nurse consultant and will need to be identified and approached. A direct approach may be effective, but there are also indirect ways for the nurse consultant to make himself or herself known to potential clients, and some client contacts may result.

For example, the nurse consultant can begin a publicity campaign to bring himself or herself to the attention of potential clients. Once the clients have been targeted, the nurse consultant does research on them: Who are they? What are they like? Where are they located? Where do they meet? What do they read? Who do they know? Once this information has been collected, the nurse consultant takes action: writing letters to the editor of publications read by the target clients; attending meetings the potential clients may also attend; becoming involved in professional or trade associations; volunteering to speak at a gathering of potential clients; becoming listed in rosters of consultants; and asking friends for introductions to potential clients they know.

The nurse consultant also may choose to work with another, already established consultant to gain entrée into the field. These arrangements should be clearly spelled out and should not turn into a situation where the nurse consultant is working *for* another individual rather than working *with* another individual. The elements that have been agreed on by both parties should be put in writing and should include specific information, such as who will perform what activities, and what benefits will accrue from the performance of those activities (whether or not the novice nurse consultant is being paid for his or her work). The agreement should include information about what will happen at the conclusion of the relationship. For example, the nurse consultant may have to sign a "no compete" agreement that specifies that he or she may not attempt to lure clients away from the other consultant, or that he or she may not consult in a specific area for a time following termination of the arrangement. (See chapter 2 for additional information on contractual arrangements.)

In developing these collaborative ventures, the nurse consultant can offer to assist the other consultant with data collection, interviews, developing proposals, or writing progress reports or final reports, to obtain experience with these aspects of consultation and to add the other consultant to the nurse consultant's network. Referrals can be obtained from these collaborative efforts, but the nurse consultant must never steal the other consultant's clients. In the event that the nurse consultant receives referrals from this colleague—or from anyone else—it is essential to acknowledge the source of the referral. Note cards that say, "Thank you for the referral" are available in office supply stores, but a handwritten note or small gift, such as flowers or candy, also is appropriate. The nurse consultant should make referrals to the other individual as well, so that there is a reciprocal exchange.

Also, the nurse consultant may accept a consulting contract that provides income but is not the consultant's primary focus. This will provide exposure to other potential clients while ensuring revenue and will also allow the consultant to gain experience. The work to be performed, however, must be within the consultant's area of expertise. If the consultant expects referrals and additional business from the project, he or she must do an excellent job. Referrals are an integral component of future business: A satisfied client refers someone else to the nurse consultant. This word-of-mouth advertising is invaluable; it cannot be bought—it must be earned, and there is no substitute for it.

Indeed, in the survey of nurse consultants conducted by the authors in mid-1995, most of the 128 respondents (81, or 63%) revealed that their most important source of referrals was clients, whereas only 30 (23%) said their most important source of referrals was other nurses.

According to Brown (1994, p. 82), the three factors that will ensure that consultants will get clients are:

1. Being known
2. Having a reputation for doing good work
3. Offering something that people need

Consultants will not be offered work if no one knows they are available and capable of doing such work. Therefore, it is imperative for the nurse consultant to market his or her services in a variety of ways.

Among the most successful methods for many consultants are making presentations to audiences composed of potential clients and writing for publication in journals read by potential clients (see the discussions below). The authors' survey of nurse consultants confirmed that these were important avenues for obtaining clients. Of 128 respondents, 44 (34%) credited speaking engagements as their most important source of referrals, and 14 (11%) credited publications. Both of these activities have the added benefit of bestowing credibility on the consultant's ideas because they are presented in a public forum.

Another activity that will result in visibility for the nurse consultant is becoming involved in professional, trade, and community organizations. Seventeen of 128 respondents (13%) in the survey of nurse consultants attributed their referrals to their activities in professional associations.

Volunteering to lead an employing institution's United Way campaign; serving on a board or committee of a community organization such as Big Brothers–Big Sisters; or assuming an elected or appointed position in a state nurses association may result in consulting opportunities, and almost certainly will result in the consultant's obtaining knowledge and skills that will pay off in the future. In the survey of nurse consultants, seven individuals (5%) said they obtained clients through their participation in committees, though only four (3%) credited social functions as an important source of referrals.

Some of these ways of finding clients can be described as indirect marketing. "Indirect" marketing is different from "direct" marketing, which is more like selling (Metzger, 1993, p. 17). The two kinds of marketing are discussed in the following sections.

INDIRECT MARKETING

Metzger (1993) describes several specific methods of indirect marketing, including the following:

1. Designing targeted research
2. Writing for publication
3. Presenting papers

4. Providing interviews
5. Writing for newspapers
6. Networking

Designing Targeted Research

Targeted research is one form of indirect marketing. Consultants can create a demand for their services by developing research projects that can be of potential use to a client group. Although much research tends to be scholarly in nature and performed in response to requirements for graduation from academic programs or promotion and tenure, research studies can be designed that will result in practical solutions to real problems. For example, the nurse consultant who studies strategic planning in associations develops a base of knowledge that can be applied to associations in a consultation arrangement. The nurse who develops an intervention in relation to a common problem experienced by a patient population and tests the intervention in a research study can use that effort in consulting with health care professionals working with the specific patient population. For example, the nurse consultant can develop a behavioral intervention for incontinence; test the intervention in a study of patients with incontinence; and then implement the intervention in health care organizations, such as long-term care facilities, where patients experience incontinence. To take another example, the nurse consultant can study the effectiveness of management techniques and as a result write, present, and consult in the arena of effective management.

An example of targeted research that has resulted in a variety of opportunities is the work of Judith Briles (1994). Briles explored the phenomenon of workplace sabotage—from withholding critical information to taking credit for someone else's work. In a nationwide study of women in the health professions, she elicited numerous examples of "unethical behavior" from individuals in randomly selected women's centers and hospitals and from members of the National Association of Women Health Professionals. Of the individuals who responded, 98% were women. Several were nurses, but the exact number is not provided. The nurses varied in educational background from those with diplomas to those with doctoral preparation.

The results of the survey indicated that most of the respondents experienced undermining of work relations on the part of another woman. One third of the respondents indicated they did not want to work with or for another woman. Respondents overwhelmingly reported, however, that they had been helped by another woman. The type of help ranged from support to mentoring. Briles also conducted interviews in which respondents were asked to describe specific incidents in which workplace sabotage occurred and to describe how the situation was resolved.

As a result of this research, Briles has appeared on television talk shows, has keynoted numerous conferences, and has published her work. Briles also has leveraged this targeted research into her practice as a management consultant who specializes in women's issues.

Writing for Publication

A second form of indirect marketing is writing for publication. Consultants can advertise their services by publishing in the field in which they wish to offer consulting services. A nurse consultant who wishes to consult in rehabilitation, therefore, would write for rehabilitation publications. Writing for publication should not be intimidating to the individual who has expertise in a field—it simply is a matter of putting that expertise in writing. What the consultant knows, however, must be applied to situations similar to those in which the consultant wishes to consult so that readers immediately recognize the applicability to their situation.

Writing for publication conveys the credibility of the consultant's ideas, particularly if the journal is peer reviewed. Writing for publication communicates a message to the readers of the publication, and according to Barnum (1995), "Having something to communicate is the first step in successful professional writing" (p. 3).

In the event that those in the consultant's audience are not readers of professional journals, then efforts must be made to publish in the periodicals read by potential clients. It may be possible to rework a professional topic into one suitable for a lay audience so that the idea is published in a scholarly journal and then in a business journal, for example.

Metzger (1993) also advises reworking the ideas of colleagues—giving necessary credit—and publishing them. The key is to publish the ideas using a pragmatic approach that will allow readers to see clearly how to apply the ideas in their own setting, thus perhaps triggering calls for the consultant's assistance.

Presenting Papers

A third kind of indirect marketing is presenting papers. The consultant also should determine what conferences are held in the field in which he or she is consulting. Most of these conferences are planned well in advance, so it is important to start early. Then the nurse consultant can contact the planners and offer his or her services as a speaker. It is critical to identify not only the professional audience—such as pediatric or rehabilitation nurses, for example—but others in the industry, such as administrators of rehabilitation facilities or physicians who specialize in pediatric rehabilitation, who might be interested in what the nurse consultant has to say.

These conferences often are advertised in the publications targeted toward the specific audiences, so the nurse consultant must read these publications on a regular basis.

Some conference planners may be reluctant to schedule a speaker whom they do not know. Therefore, the nurse consultant should be prepared to offer references who will attest to his or her abilities. If possible, an audiotape or a videotape of a previous presentation should be available to send to the sponsor. The nurse consultant also may want to develop and maintain a list of presentations, including information such as date of the presentation, topic, sponsor, size of audience, and relevant evaluative comments. This list will serve two purposes: It can be used as a reminder when answering a sponsor's specific questions about presentation history, and it can be used as a marketing device in apprising sponsors of other topics that the nurse consultant may address.

Responding to a "Call for Abstracts." Some conference planners obtain speakers through a "call for abstracts" process rather than through invitations. In that case, the nurse consultant needs to respond to the call as specified by the conference sponsors. Pierce and Gregg (1994) identified the following elements of an abstract:

1. Cover page, which includes identifying information about the presenter (e.g., name, credentials, place of employment, address, and telephone number)
2. Body of the abstract, which includes the following:
   - Purpose of the presentation
   - Relation to the conference theme
   - Objectives
   - Summary of the presentation
   - Implications for practice
   - Selected readings

The request for presentations may also include instructions about submitting a curriculum vitae or résumé, references from previous speaking engagements, or other information about the presentation or presenter. It is necessary to comply exactly with the submission requirements. It is important to tailor the abstract according to the directions provided by the sponsor; abstracts that do not conform generally are not even reviewed.

In addition, the nurse consultant should

1. Use keywords from the call, such as those in the conference theme and goals
2. Focus on the target audience

3. Relate the content of the response to the level of the audience (i.e., basic, intermediate, or advanced practitioners in the field)

Preparing for a Presentation.   Once the presentation has been selected, more work must be done. In preparing for the presentation, the nurse consultant should

1. Speak with someone who has presented to this audience before
2. Review abstracts of presentations at a previous conference
3. Purchase a tape of a presentation at a previous conference
4. Talk with someone who has attended a previous conference

The sponsor of the conference may be willing to provide this information to the nurse consultant on request. If not, it may be necessary to obtain the information from other contacts. Although this may seem to be a great deal of work for just one presentation, the fact that potential clients may be in the audience should make the effort worthwhile.

Metzger (1993) proposes that the consultant be "able to deliver a solid talk that provides practical new insights and advice" (p. 25) as a way of generating consultation offers from the audience. If the presentation is successful, there is every likelihood that the nurse consultant will be contacted by others in the industry and invited to speak again. Metzger (pp. 26–27) offers these tips for successful presentations to an audience of potential clients:

- Strive to reach small audiences (volunteer for a concurrent rather than a plenary session) in order to have the intimacy needed to sell the consultant's services effectively.
- Know who is in the audience in order to be able to tailor remarks to the audience.
- Present only a few key points and then reinforce them throughout the presentation (tell the audience what you are going to say, then say it, and then close by telling the audience what you just said).
- Identify with the audience, whether it consists of professionals or laypeople; use "we."
- Speak for less than the allotted time, to allow for questions and answers. This will permit members of the audience to inquire about specific problems that the consultant then can address, thus marketing his or her services to specific individuals.
- Try to be scheduled early in the conference—preferably in the morning, before lunch.
- Do not start or end the presentation with a joke; the audience wants to hear new and practical ideas, not humor.

Although Metzger (1993) recommends not telling jokes, other noted consultants (Holtz, 1993) suggest that humor is generally well accepted. Still, unless the speaker is adept in telling a joke or story, it is better not to attempt one.

In addition, it is helpful for the speaker to always include at least one idea that the audience can take home and apply immediately. For example, in addressing a group of Girl Scout leaders on getting and keeping volunteer troop leaders, the speaker may describe how the job can be shared between two adults and then demonstrate exactly how to accomplish this goal.

The dilemma here is maintaining the delicate balance between providing value for the audience and not giving away information for which the consultant rightly should be paid. One means of ensuring that materials will not be used without the consultant's knowledge is to copyright them. For example, a nurse consultant who prepares a workshop on violence in the workplace develops a package consisting of a content outline, references and resources, handouts, transparencies, and a script. Someone could take these materials and present the workshop on his or her own if the workshop package was not copyrighted. Similarly, a consultant might prepare an outline detailing the steps involved in an executive search, which if not copyrighted could be used by anyone without the consultant's knowledge or permission.

Although this kind of unethical activity seldom occurs, the nurse can file for copyright protection of his or her products by filing an application with the Registrar of Copyrights, Library of Congress, Washington, DC 20559. A small fee is charged for filing.

Understanding Public Speaking. Public speaking is an excellent medium for conveying a consultant's message to the appropriate target audience. Unfortunately, many people are afraid to speak in public. Knowledge about the elements of public speaking and extensive preparation, however, can do much to dispel this fear.

Klarman and Mateo (1994, pp. 307–308) offer information about the five basic elements of public speaking:

1. Message
2. Purpose
3. Speaker
4. Audience
5. Situation

Message. The message of a presentation can be conveyed if the speaker follows the "tell them" formula: tell them what you are going to tell them; tell them; and then tell them what you told them. Writing the message in a simple, declarative sentence before preparing the presentation will keep the message clear and focused.

Purpose.   The purpose of the presentation should coincide with one of the four basic purposes of public speaking: (1) to inform, (2) to persuade, (3) to inspire, (4) to entertain. In the case of the nurse consultant making a presentation, the primary purpose will generally be to inform the audience about a specific topic but the secondary purpose will be to persuade at least some of the audience members to subsequently avail themselves of the consultant's services.

Speaker.   The speaker must be prepared to address the specific topic. Experience in public speaking is desirable for nurse consultants, but until the nurse consultant can accumulate this experience, practice in front of a mirror or, preferably, in front of colleagues can suffice.

An effective way to practice and improve speaking skills is to join Toastmasters International, an organization with branches in many cities. In Toastmasters meetings members make impromptu speeches, which then are critiqued. Many noted individuals credit Toastmasters for their success in public speaking (Mackay, 1992).

Successful speakers cultivate a style of presentation that complements their personality. Two styles suggested by Hoff (1992) are "blue-zone"and "red-zone" speakers. Blue-zone speakers present topics in a logical, organized, intellectual style. Red-zone speakers often speak extemporaneously, and their presentations are characterized by an impulsive, emotional style. Neither zone is preferable over the other; to become an accomplished speaker, the nurse consultant must be aware of his or her presentation characteristics and use them effectively in relation to the purpose of the speech.

Bedrosian (1987) provides a means of assessing a speaker's presentation style in terms of the following characteristics: "detailed, organized, logical, intuitive, action-oriented, and spontaneous" (p. 34). Although these characteristics will vary depending on other aspects of the presentation—such as the audience and the content of the speech—each has advantages and disadvantages that the nurse consultant should be aware of in developing and using a speaking style.

Audience.   Successful speakers know as much about the audience to whom they are speaking as they know about the topic. Familiarity with the audience will help the nurse consultant tailor the presentation to the concerns of the audience, considering such factors as education, employment, age, gender, reasons for being in the audience, and others. Stone and Bachner (1977) suggest that asking for a liaison person from the audience to be addressed will help ensure a successful presentation, as long as the liaison is truly representative of the potential audience. They further suggest several questions for the liaison to help the speaker prepare for the presentation. Among the questions to ask are the following:

1. What is the occasion for the presentation?
2. What is the speaker expected to talk about?
3. What does the audience already know about the topic?
4. What is the age range, economic status, and educational level of the audience?

Another strategy is to interview three to four individuals who will be in the audience. The sponsor of the event at which the presentation will occur will be able to supply the names of possible audience representatives. The nurse consultant then can ask questions such as the following:

1. What are common concerns about the topic?
2. What strategies have been used to deal with situations, problems, or issues related to the topic?
3. What kind of information on the topic is the audience looking for?

The presentation then can be based on this information. During the presentation, the nurse consultant may wish to acknowledge the assistance of the audience representatives by saying, "I've spoken with several of you before this presentation and have learned that your most common concern about the topic is . . ." The speaker may wish to acknowledge the audience representatives by name, but it is wise to check with them beforehand if naming them publicly might embarrass them or make them uncomfortable in any way.

Situation. The final factor to consider is the situation: time of day, location, and the length of the presentation. A lunch speaker uses a different style from a banquet speaker, and a keynote speech differs from one given in a concurrent session. The location of the presentation may determine whether audiovisual aids can be used, and the length of the presentation affects how much information can be conveyed.

Speaking to a professional audience does not differ much from speaking to industry executives; however, the nurse consultant may be more comfortable with the former audience because of his or her level of familiarity with them. To familiarize himself or herself with an audience, the nurse consultant can review the literature in the industry, attend social or educational events in the industry, and talk with contacts in his or her network who are in the industry. Working with audience representatives or a liaison from the industry is essential in this instance.

Providing Interviews

A fourth type of indirect marketing is giving interviews. Metzger (1993) suggests that as the consultant's work gets transmitted via publications and presentations, the consultant will be approached by the media to discuss his or her ideas. Vogel and Doleysh (1994) note that this publicity usually is free and has the added benefit of enhancing the consultant's credibility.

Metzger also suggests ways to inform the media of the importance of the consultant's contributions—for example, press releases. Press releases should actually be used to announce significant events, such as the outcomes of a research project, rather than to announce a presentation to be made by the nurse consultant. Other means exist to publicize the activities of the nurse consultant. Newsletters of professional and trade associations and alumni organizations often include "members' news," and the consultant can submit frequent items to these publications. Some professional journals also publish information on new products, services, or information. The nurse consultant should carefully target the appropriate publications for announcements about his or her activities; it is a waste of time and money for both the consultant and the recipient when communications are transmitted needlessly.

A media interview offers the nurse consultant another opportunity to market his or her services and should be planned as carefully as a presentation before an audience at a conference. Identify two or three points, and make those the focal point of the interview. Reinforce the points with examples that illustrate the application to the desired audience. For example, a nurse consultant who has developed a program informing employers and employees about sexual harassment in the workplace might stress (1) the need for employers to develop guidelines describing what constitutes sexual harassment in a particular workplace, (2) the ways in which sexual harassment can be identified by the employee, and (3) the joint responsibility of employee and employer to resolve any complaints of sexual harassment. These three points as the focus of a media interview will reach both employees and employers watching the program.

Writing for Newspapers

A fifth form of indirect marketing is writing for newspapers. Newspapers, particularly weekly, community, or business journals, like all publications, look for material that is relevant to readers. The nurse consultant can write an opinion piece about the results of research that are relevant to a lay audience. The contribution should be brief and to the point, and written for people with an eighth-grade reading level.

Metzger, an expert in business policy, wrote a monthly column on marketing strategy targeted toward bankers, his primary clients. Although a great deal of time is required to develop a relationship with a newspaper's editors that will culminate in such an opportunity, nonetheless appearing in print periodically will provide a public relations boost to any consultant's business.

Networking

Finally, a sixth form of indirect marketing is networking. Metzger (1993) further describes as sources of referrals individuals in the same professional and social associations as the consultant. A variety of networking strategies can be used to promote the consultant's services (see chapter 7).

DIRECT MARKETING

Direct marketing is a sales effort targeted toward marketing the consultant's services to potential clients. Various strategies constitute direct marketing, among them "cold" calling, responding to "requests for proposals" (RFPs), and direct mail campaigns. In general, direct marketing is more difficult than indirect marketing because it involves proactive selling. It often is viewed as a "commercial" activity, but it is one in which the consultant must engage if he or she wishes to maintain existing clients and expand the business.

As long as the direct marketing efforts are conducted professionally and ethically, there will be no adverse reaction to them. According to Levinson (1993), honesty is a golden rule in marketing. Levinson adds that "dishonesty is one of the mortal enemies of your reputation and your marketing" (p. 45).

A Six-Step Letter Campaign

Metzger (1993, pp. 36–40)) describes one way of getting clients through direct marketing, which he says has been successful for him: developing a letter campaign. The six steps of the campaign are as follows:

1. Select an industry
2. Develop a mailing list
3. Develop an issues letter
4. Mail 10 letters a week
5. Follow up with telephone calls
6. Conduct sales calls

Each of these steps is explained briefly below.

Step 1: Select an Industry.   Initially, the consultant must decide on which industry to focus the marketing efforts. The selection depends on the consultant's area of expertise. For the nurse consultant, the industry may be nursing, health care, or perhaps nursing associations or health care associations. The next step involves identifying the two or three issues that are critical to the profession at the time. The consultant's premise about the critical issues should be verified with leaders in the field. Research in the local library also can help confirm the validity of the critical issues. Perhaps the consultant is a nursing staff development educator who identifies two critical issues: (1) the lack of documented evidence of the impact of continuing education on the subsequent practice of nurses, and (2) the restructuring of staff development departments in health care facilities from centralized to decentralized and from a focus on nursing-specific education to hospitalwide education. These issues can be validated through a review of the literature in the field; conversations with other nursing staff development educators; and discussions with leaders of organized groups of nursing staff development educators, such as the National Nursing Staff Development Organization (NNSDO) or the American Nurses Association Council for Professional Nursing Education and Development. In this example, the nursing staff development consultant may discover that the first issue (the impact of continuing education on nursing practice) is a formidable one for which many institutions may not have the resources to support exploration, and may thus decide to focus instead on the second issue—restructuring.

Step 2: Develop a Mailing List.   Next, the consultant develops a mailing list of organizations that will be affected by the critical issues in the industry, beginning with those closest to home and working outward in concentric circles. The mailing list should include the name and title of the decision maker in the organization. In the example above, the staff development consultant may target large hospitals in medical centers as well as in rural settings.

Step 3: Develop an Issues Letter.   The consultant then drafts a letter to the decision maker in the targeted organizations. This letter is for the purpose of obtaining an interview to discuss the critical issues facing the decision maker. In the example given, the letter might be sent to the chief executive officer (CEO) as well as to the head of the staff development department in the institution.

The letter should clearly indicate that the consultant is knowledgeable about this critical issue facing the industry through both education and experiential background and, furthermore, may be able to assist the decision maker in dealing with this critical issue. The approach should not be a "hard sell" at this point, because the letter is intended only to introduce the consultant to the decision maker.

Step 4: Mail 10 Letters a Week. Metzger (1993) suggests sending only a few letters each week, because each letter must be followed by a telephone call. Mailing to a large list at one time means that many telephone calls will need to be made, and given the difficulty of reaching some people, may require more time than the consultant is able to devote without adversely affecting his or her workload.

Step 5: Follow Up with Telephone Calls. Each letter should be followed by a telephone call to obtain an appointment with the decision maker. In dealing with individuals who screen calls for the decision maker, it is important to be pleasant but persistent. It may be difficult to reach the person to whom the letter was addressed, but it is essential to make an appointment with the person most likely to be in a position to engage the consultant's services. If necessary after numerous calls, fax a copy of the original letter with a handwritten note on the bottom describing unsuccessful attempts to reach the decision maker; that strategy may trigger a response, if only because the decision maker realizes that the consultant will continue to be persistent.

Step 6: Conduct Sales Calls. Metzger (1993) states that one interview will result from every 10 letters sent. He describes his own experiences in generating business, in which 110 letters, followed by 680 telephone calls, resulted in 21 appointments and 3 consultation contracts. Metzger asserts that this approach will result in business.

The interviews generated by the letter campaign represent a difficult part of the direct marketing effort. Initially, the nurse consultant establishes rapport with the potential client: He or she thanks the individual for the opportunity to meet, describes his or her work and area of expertise as it applies to the potential client, and then focuses the remainder of the conversation on the client.

In the interviews, the goal is to elicit the client's problem. This is best accomplished by asking a series of general questions, such as: "What is going well for you? What is not going well? Why or why not?" During this general discussion, the client will have an opportunity to discuss successes; after sharing what has worked, a natural progression into difficulties and problems will occur. Then, narrow the scope of the interview to determine the real problem.

Ask more specific questions, such as: "Who else agrees that this is a problem?" "How have you tried to solve this problem?" At this point in the interview, the nurse consultant should have an idea about what he or she might be able to offer the client. This critical point is where the nurse consultant must sell his or her services. Ask a question such as: "May I prepare a proposal to work with you in resolving this issue?" The answer may be yes, but according to Metzger (1993), statistically speaking, about 4 of 5 times it will not be yes, for a variety of reasons.

If the answer is no, after an attempt is made to determine the reasons for saying no and attempting to overcome the objections, the consultant should thank the decision maker for his or her time and leave. It is advisable to write a thank-you note, again stressing appreciation for the time spent and suggesting that the consultant may be of service in the future.

If, however, this is the one time in five that the response is affirmative, follow up with a question about the process for approving such a proposal. The response to this question will provide useful information about who else in the organization will be involved and whom the consultant must also meet or influence to obtain the contract for the project. The decision maker is likely to reveal this information when asked general questions, such as: "Who else will be involved in this project?" "What will be the person's role?" "What will be the individual's interest in the project?"

Following completion of this step, the consultant prepares the proposal, dealing specifically with the interests of all parties potentially involved in the project. For example, if the CEO and the chief financial officer both will be involved, the proposal must address the salient financial matters as well as the administrative concerns. See chapter 4 for a description of how to prepare and present a proposal to a client to win the business.

Additional Strategies of Direct Marketing

A variety of other ways of direct marketing also exist, among them the following (Cohen, 1991):

- Direct mail
- Cold calls
- Advertising
- Directory listings
- Former employers

Each of these marketing strategies is described briefly below.

Direct Mail.   In a direct mailing, the consultant sends potential clients a letter, a brochure, or other written materials to advertise his or her services. As described above with regard to Metzger's letter campaign, the purpose of the direct mailing is to establish communication with the potential client. Thus, direct mail must address the perceived needs of the client for the consultant's services and convince the client that the consultant is the appropriate individual to meet those needs. The way a direct mailing is written is key to whether it is read by the recipient.

The piece must be attractive enough to get the reader's attention. The first paragraph in a direct mail letter must interest the client enough to keep him or her reading. Cohen (1991) suggests identifying several accomplishments and then selecting one that illustrates the results of the consultant's work. This accomplishment would form the first paragraph, such as: "Your colleague Mary Smith, from Memorial Hospital, just called to thank me for helping them prepare for a Joint Commission survey. She was excited because for the first time in the hospital's history they received accreditation with commendation—and she attributed it to me!"

Such an opening is guaranteed to attract attention and encourage the recipient to read further. In the succeeding text, the consultant states the purpose of the letter, as "I am writing because I consult with agencies that are seeking accreditation by the Joint Commission on Accreditation of Healthcare Organizations (JCAHO). If you are interested in saving time and money in preparing for a survey, you may be interested to know that I . . ." Here the consultant lists accomplishments related to working with other clients seeking JCAHO accreditation. This listing should be brief and to the point; quantify accomplishments wherever possible. The potential client thus realizes that what the consultant has done for others could also be done for him or her.

If possible, include in the direct mailing piece testimonials from previous clients. Verbatim remarks are best, but permission must be obtained to use them. If you do not have permission, paraphrase the remark and attribute it to a position, such as "staff development director, medical center hospital of 1,000 beds."

Educational background of the consultant may be included if it is relevant to the potential project. Experience with similar projects must be included. A brief statement should suffice, such as: "I have a master's degree in nursing from the University of Iowa and a doctorate in organizational development from Harvard. I have been consulting in health care for more than 15 years." If space allows, the consultant can list other clients.

Conclude the direct mailing with a call to action. The client should be asked to call or write for further information about the nurse consultant's services. Directions about the expected action should be clear and explicit.

Cohen (1991) recommends closing the letter with a postscript (P.S.), which is almost always read, sometimes even before the recipient reads the rest of the letter. The P.S. should be used to further stimulate the desired action. Cohen further suggests that the consultant offer something free in exchange for the action, such as: "If you call or write, I will send you a complimentary reprint of my article, "Preparing for JCAHO Can Be

Fun—and Effective!" which appeared in the *National Nursing Journal* in
May this year. Call or write today, while copies last."

The letter should be printed on the consultant's letterhead and should be
no more than one page in length. The letter should be addressed to an individual by name, and should be free of grammatical or typographical errors.

A brochure rather than a letter can be used, but a brochure is less personal than a letter. A brochure can accompany a personal letter, however.
The letter, the brochure, or both should include a business card (see chapters 5 and 7 for information on business cards). The purpose of a brochure
is to answer two questions: "What is it that I do?" and "Why am I the best?"
(Cohen, 1991).

The brochure can include information on specific services provided by
the consultant, previous and current clients, statements of satisfaction
from clients, special qualifications and accomplishments, and a description
of the consultant's background. The basic contents of a brochure include
"who you are, what you do, how you work, what you've done, and how
to contact you" (Cohen, 1991, pp. 29–30).

The brochure should be professionally designed and printed. Many
computer software programs exist that allow users to incorporate graphics
with text, but care must be taken that the results of using such a program
do not appear amateurish. The time and money invested in developing a
brochure generally are substantial, so it is worthwhile to make every effort
to produce a professional result that will reflect well on the consultant and
generate business opportunities.

However, it is imperative to remember that what the brochure or letter
says is more important to the potential client than how it looks. The purpose of the design is only to capture the attention of the potential client
long enough to encourage him or her to read; the content, not the design,
of the brochure will generate the business.

It is important to proofread the brochure numerous times before it is
printed. Individuals in addition to the consultant should be engaged to
review the brochure for content as well as layout. Individuals representing previous clients can provide valuable feedback on the aspects of the
brochure that are most appealing to potential clients.

The brochure must then be mailed to the appropriate audience for the
consultant's services. The consultant should develop the mailing list by
determining potential clients for the specific services offered. Commercial
companies provide mailing lists, but these generally are not targeted specifically enough for the nurse consultant's purposes, and they often are "rent-
ed" rather than sold, so that the list may be used only for a one-time mailing.

Compiling the mailing list is labor intensive, but once developed the
list can be used for follow-up mailings as well. For this reason, it is best
to enter the mailing list into a computer program, either a database or

word-processing program, so that it can be changed, modified, and retrieved at will.

The mailing list should be targeted toward potential clients who are most likely to use the consultant's services. Because of the cost of preparing, printing, and mailing direct mail pieces (letter or brochure), it makes sense not to waste money on those who have only a slight likelihood of being interested in the services being marketed.

A caveat is necessary here. The consultant may consider adding to the direct mailing a trinket, such as a pen, a notepad, or some other item with his or her name on it, in the hope of garnering business by having the consultant's name in front of the potential client whenever the item is used. It probably is wiser to focus on the content of the direct mailing to ensure that it meets the needs of potential clients, rather than providing a novelty item. These novelty items can be expensive and often are duplicated by many others seeking the same business. Unless the nurse consultant can afford to dispense a valuable item, such as a desk clock or a crystal paperweight, omit these gifts.

Cold Calls.   Cold calls are difficult to make, because they can result in rejection, but, according to Cohen (1991), they also are effective in getting business. In using this technique, the nurse consultant first targets potential clients and sets a goal for calling efforts—perhaps 20 calls in one day. If just one of the calls results in a contract for services, the effort will have been worthwhile. Cohen (1991) says that cold calling will be more successful if the consultant

- Prepares a script for the call, which follows the outline of the direct mailing
- Uses creative ways to avoid having the call screened: for instance, by calling before 8 A.M. or after 5 P.M., when the target client may be in the office but the secretary may not
- Realizes that a successful cold call results in an interview, not a sale
- Combines cold calls with direct mail by sending the mail piece first and following up with a call several weeks later

Advertising.   The nurse consultant may choose to advertise his or her services in professional or trade publications. However, the respondents in the survey of nurse consultants conducted by the authors in mid-1995 did not rank advertising as an important source of referrals; only 10 of 128 respondents (8%) said they obtained clients through advertisements.

If this means of obtaining clients is used, it is imperative that the advertisement be well written—targeted toward an audience of potential clients. Because advertising is expensive, it is necessary to target carefully the places in which such advertising may appear. Following the outline for the direct mailing described above will ensure that the advertisement meets the needs of the appropriate group.

The advertisement also needs to be professionally prepared. Many quick-print shops employ individuals who can lay out an advertisement and produce it through typesetting or a desktop publishing program on a computer. This "camera-ready" art then is sent to the publication. The printer can produce multiple copies; it is the initial preparation that is expensive—additional copies do not add substantially to the cost.

Directory Listings. The consultant may wish to consider advertising in specialized publications, such as the *Women's Yellow Pages,* now appearing in many cities; or in listings of consultants, such as the "Directory of Nurse Consultants" that appears biannually in the *Journal of Nursing Administration* (JONA). Listings in the JONA Directory are $100 each, and consultants can purchase additional space for a display advertisement. Listings of consultants also appear on the World Wide Web and can be accessed through the Internet.

Directory listings, however, are generally not very effective. Most clients do not consult them when attempting to locate a consultant—they rely on other means, such as referrals or recommendations from others—word-of-mouth. Before investing a great deal of money in such advertising, the nurse consultant may wish to test a specific directory for a year or so to determine how effective it is in generating business.

Former Employers. Cohen (1991) suggests that many consultants obtain their initial work by consulting with former employers who are familiar with the consultant's skills and who gain by not having to pay the consultant a salary and other benefits, such as health insurance. Often, the consultant can command a higher rate as a consultant than he or she enjoyed as an employee. The former employer then can serve as a valuable reference for the nurse consultant for future opportunities.

MARKETING TO PREVIOUS CLIENTS

One often neglected aspect of identifying the target audience and developing marketing strategies to reach that audience is including former clients as part of the target audience. It is generally well known that small businesses often neglect their previous clients, and most nursing consultation practices are small businesses. It is essential to include previous clients in the customer base; after all, they have provided business to the nurse consultant in the past and, if they were satisfied, are likely to do so again in the future.

Marketing to past clients should include an incentive for their future business. Like the car-wash company that offers the tenth wash free after nine have been purchased, or the airline programs that offer frequent-flier benefits to build customers' loyalty, the nurse consultant may consider offering a special enticement for repeat clients.

A consultant who specializes in accreditation of continuing education programs may keep track of the accreditation period for associations with whom she has consulted. Then, as the time to submit an application for accreditation nears, she contacts the organization and offers to assist in the preparation of the application and cites a reduced fee because the organization is a previous client.

It is also important to remember that organizations today are outsourcing tasks and activities that constitute only part of a job. Opportunities abound for taking advantage of these outsourcing thrusts. If the consultant is willing to undertake the registration process for a conference rather than manage the entire conference, there may be work available. Lobbying, record keeping, and education targeted toward meeting the requirements of regulatory agencies are a few of the activities being outsourced. The savvy consultant will market services for these parts of a project as well as for the project in its entirety.

SUMMARY

Although marketing may not be an activity with which nurses are comfortable—or even familiar—it is an essential component of a nurse consultant's repertoire of skills. Sources for learning about marketing abound; in addition to the numerous texts on the subject, community colleges often give continuing education courses that address public relations skills. Small-business development centers in colleges and universities also help individuals learn to market their businesses. Credit courses in business administration departments in colleges often welcome the noncredit student. Noncredit students bring an outside perspective to their studies that can benefit all of the students enrolled in a class. Thus, while the nurse consultant is learning marketing, he or she can be providing valuable perspectives to fellow students—and making valuable contacts in the process.

Not knowing how to market should not be a deterrent to becoming a consultant, but it is as important to learn marketing skills as it is to develop expertise in a specific area in which the consultant wishes to offer his or her services. A marketing effort that is well planned and well implemented will help the nurse consultant identify and generate clients, forecast trends and issues in the field that may affect the services the nurse consultant offers, set reasonable fees, and know about and deal with competition for his or her services. Simply stated, marketing effectively is a key not only to the start-up of a consulting venture but also to its growth and development.

REFERENCES

Alward, R. R., & Camuñas, C. (1991). *The nurse's guide to marketing*. Albany, NY: Delmar.

Barnum, B. S. (1995). *Writing and getting published*. New York: Springer.

Bedrosian, M. M. (1987). *Speak like a pro*. New York: John Wiley & Sons.

Briles, J. (1994). *The Briles report on women in health care*. San Francisco: Jossey-Bass.

Brown, P. C. (1994). *Jumping the job track: Security, satisfaction, and success as an independent consultant*. New York: Crown.

Cohen, W. A. (1991). *How to make it big as a consultant* (2nd ed.). New York: AMA-COM.

Drucker, P. (1973). *The practice of management*. New York: Harper & Row.

Echeveste, D. W. (1982). Marketing and business. In B. R. Riccardi & E. C. Dayani (Eds.), *The nurse entrepreneur* (pp. 43–62). Reston, VA: Reston.

Ethier, D. (1988). Marketing. In H. Ernstthal & V. Jefferson (Eds.), *Principles of association management* (2nd ed., pp. 107–113). Washington, DC: American Society of Association Executives.

Hoff, R. (1992). *I can see you naked: A fearless guide to making great presentations*. New York: Andrews & McNeel.

Holtz, H. (1983). *How to succeed as an independent consultant*. New York: John Wiley & Sons.

Holtz, H. (1992). *The consultant's guide to hidden profits*. New York: John Wiley & Sons.

Holtz, H. (1993). *How to succeed as an independent consultant* (3rd ed.). New York: John Wiley & Sons.

Kelly, K. J. (1987). Marketing. In B. E. Puetz, *Contemporary strategies for continuing education in nursing* (pp. 187–217). Rockville, MD: Aspen.

Klarman, K. L., & Mateo, M. A. (1994). An approach to presentation skill development of nurses. *Journal of Nursing Staff Development, 10,* 307–311.

Levinson, J. C. (1993). *Guerrilla marketing excellence*. Boston: Houghton Mifflin.

Mackay, H. (Speaker). (1992). *Sharkproof* (cassette recording). New York: HarperCollins.

Metzger, R. O. (1993). *Developing a consulting practice*. Newbury Park, CA: Sage.

Stone, J., & Bachner, J. (1977). *Speaking up*. New York: McGraw-Hill.

Vogel, G., & Doleysh, N. (1994). *Entrepreneuring: A nurse's guide to starting a business* (2nd ed.). New York: National League for Nursing Press.

7

Networking

Networking is an integral component of success in consultation. Getting started, finding clients, marketing services, making the business grow, and being successful all depend in large part on the networking skills of the nurse consultant. In this chapter, the process of making and using contacts to progress in a career path, and the accoutrements of networking, such as business cards, are described. In addition, specific strategies for increasing success in networking are noted.

DEFINITIONS OF NETWORKING

The author of the seminal work on networking defined it as "the process of developing and using your contacts for information, advice and moral support as you pursue your career" (Welch, 1980, p. 15). According to Fisher and Vilas (1992), networking is "making links from people we know to people they know, in an organized way, for a specific purpose, while remaining committed to doing our part, expecting nothing in return" (p. 8).

These authors and others describe the tangible benefits of networking, such as referrals, business, information, and advice (Hauter, 1993; Puetz, 1983, 1991, 1993; Stern, 1981; Zagury, 1993). Other, less obvious benefits of networking are the feeling of accomplishment when an individual has an opportunity to reciprocate with advice, information, a referral, or a business opportunity. Networking often builds self-esteem as well. When others seek advice, information, or referrals from us, it makes us feel better about ourselves and the contributions we can make.

Networking relies on contacts. Contacts are people from whom an individual can obtain advice, information, or business. For the nurse consultant, individuals in professional as well as personal networks are an ideal source of referrals for business opportunities. Contacts in networks can help the nurse consultant get clients and market the consultant's services to potential clients.

In some networks, members barter their products and services. For example, the Business Exchange International (BXI), located in Overland Park, Kansas, has more than 35,000 members nationwide. These individuals are in all types of businesses—from hotels to home repair to restaurants. Members barter both products and services through a monthly newsletter.

In other networks, such as the Business Network International, with chapters primarily in large metropolitan areas, individuals meet for the sole purpose of developing profitable business relationships. Often these groups limit membership to only a few in each industry (e.g., attorneys, stockbrokers, and nurses) so that one profession does not dominate.

Kelly and Joel (1995) describe another type of network: a subgroup in a nursing organization composed of nurses with common interests. Often called special interest groups, these subgroups exist to support members, share information, notify each other of job opportunities, and refer each other for professional opportunities.

Networking works as individuals exchange ideas, information, and advice. The individual seeking the information or advice had a specific purpose in mind and very likely benefited from the exchange. The individual offering the information or advice probably benefited as well, in being able to be of assistance to someone. In networking, individuals also counsel, coach, and act as mentors. In consultation, networking may result in recommendations, referrals, or other business opportunities.

IDENTIFYING NETWORKS

Networking wisdom suggests that the nurse consultant include in his or her networks people who are less experienced, people at his or her own level (colleagues and peers), and people who are more experienced (Puetz, 1983; Smith, 1993). The first group are those who will learn from the nurse consultant—those the nurse consultant will nurture and mentor. The nurse consultant's colleagues and peers form the nurse consultant's support group, and the older, wiser individuals are those whom the nurse consultant will seek as mentors. Although it is nice, and certainly advantageous, to include the "stars" in a business or industry in a professional or personal network, it is not necessary. The nurse consultant can accomplish a great deal without their assistance, and when he or she does well, the stars will want to be part of the nurse consultant's network.

Initially, to identify networks it is important to make lists of individuals who are in the three areas described above: the vertical, downward network (less experienced individuals); the horizontal network (peers or colleagues); and the vertical, upward network (more experienced persons). The lists should include those individuals with whom the nurse consultant currently is in contact and others, such as former employers and coworkers. Often, contact with the latter group has been diminished or lost over time. In this case, the nurse consultant must determine how effective it would be to reestablish contact in the hope of adding these individuals to an existing network.

The list of individuals in a network should include those in the nurse consultant's professional circle but others as well. Individuals who are in health care-related professions or with whom the consultant does business in other ways (e.g., attorneys, accountants, and members of the chamber of commerce) should be listed.

Once these contacts have been identified, the nurse consultant must make an effort to categorize them in relation to their position in the three networks described above. Their placement in the three networks will illustrate the nurse consultant's relationship with them. For example, it is possible that the nurse consultant spends a great deal of time advising, coaching, and otherwise assisting individuals in his or her vertical, downward network—perhaps even neglecting other, more productive or profitable activities as a result. To take another example, the consultant may spend time with colleagues in the horizontal network engaged in gossip or idle conversation, neither of which will accomplish any business purpose.

NETWORKING EFFECTIVELY

To network effectively, the nurse consultant must follow the "rules." First, know what the networking should accomplish—the specific *purpose* for networking. Then, develop *strategies* about whom the nurse consultant needs to know to get what is wanted or needed, and how to meet these people. For example, if the nurse consultant's networking goal is to obtain financing for a business start-up, then a meeting attended by bankers in the community is an obvious choice. Consider a chamber of commerce meeting or a workshop on "Starting a Business." Attend those meetings— as many as necessary until relationships with the appropriate people are established. The savvy nurse consultant will make an effort to maintain these relationships over time as well. Several important aspects of effective networking are discussed below.

Organizing Networks

Networking efforts must be organized; not every contact will be helpful. The Pareto principle, commonly known as the 80/20 rule (see chapter 9), applies here, as in many other situations: 80% of the results will come from 20% of the contacts. Figuring out exactly how to use contacts most effectively will make the most efficient use of the 20%.

Organizing and keeping track of contacts can be expedited by using a system such as business cards, a Rolodex file, or a computer software program. The setup of these systems is similar; they all provide a means of keeping track of names and other important information about contacts.

When information about a potential contact is received, it can be organized in one of several ways to allow the nurse consultant to easily retrieve the information. For example, a nurse consultant who receives several business cards at an educational event may write on the back of each the location of the meeting and something about the individual represented by the card, as well as any follow-up the consultant promised. The cards can be sorted by the name of the meeting; the individual's name; or topic heading, such as continuing educator, researcher, grants writer; or area of practice, such as pediatrics, home care, or oncology. In some cases, it may be necessary to classify an individual into more than one category: by area of interest for a potential consultation proposal, and by location of the conference if the nurse consultant plans to attend similar conferences in the future and can look up the contact.

Business Cards

The nurse consultant must have business cards to exchange. Business cards are an important part of networking. Business cards reflect the individual, so care must be taken that the cards project an appropriate, professional image of the consultant and his or her business (see chapter 5).

The paper on which the cards are printed should be a good-quality card stock. Ink color should be black or dark blue. It is important to avoid the temptation to design a card that will stand out from others because of vivid colors, a splashy logo, or the like; the idea is to impress clients with skills and abilities, not with the color or design of a business card.

The business card should contain the following information about the nurse consultant:

- *Name.* The full name should be used. A nickname or a preferred name by which to be addressed should be included in parentheses (e.g., Sandra A. [Sandy] Miller). Titles, such as Ms., Mr., Mrs., or Dr., should not be used with the consultant's name.
- *Credentials.* According to the *ANA Manual of Style* (3rd ed.) (American Nurses Association, 1978) the name is "followed by abbreviations . . . in sequence . . . as follows: orders, religious first; academic degrees earned in course; honorary degrees in order of bestowal; professional or occupational title. Only the highest earned

degree should be listed" (p. 18) (e.g., PhD, RN; MSEd, RN, C; DNSc, RN, FAAN).

- *Business location.* Include address with zip code and telephone number with area code. The business card also may include a fax number and an e-mail address.
- *Description of services offered.* This addition to a business card is important for a nurse consultant whose business name may not reflect his or her practice. For example, one of the authors does business under the name of Puetz & Associates, Inc. Her business card indicates that the business comprises "association management, consultation, education, and publishing."

If the information described above should change, it is necessary to print new cards. Writing on business cards to correct or change information does not give a good impression, so the cost of printing new cards when information about the consultant changes is worthwhile.

Business cards are printed inexpensively by "quick print" shops. Including a logo on the card or printing with more than one color increases the cost—sometimes substantially.

Follow-Up

Follow-up with contacts is important; it is essential to keep in touch with them. Deep and Sussman (1990) suggest sending personal notes to colleagues who have accomplished something, such as publishing a book, a chapter in a book, or an article; made a presentation; or otherwise achieved something noteworthy. Information about these accomplishments can be found in newsletters of professional and trade associations, or from contacts in conversations.

Other ways to keep in touch involve sending notices of position changes, mailing postcards from conventions that the contact had previously attended, and sending clips from newspapers or articles on topics of interest to the contact.

Finally, offer the nurse consultant's help. Is there something the nurse consultant can do in exchange for the services he or she is seeking? People tend to remember helpful individuals.

Being Gracious

Smith (1995) offers advice to individuals who wish to network effectively: Never fail to be gracious. Smith suggests that effective networkers:

- Have an attitude of "How can I help you?" Gracious individuals do not focus exclusively on what they will get from networking but rather focus on the other individual. So these gracious people are not scanning those who enter a room, trying to see if someone more important is arriving.

- Do not focus on their own self-importance. Gracious networkers do not act as if they are the most important people in the room. They introduce themselves in a way that encourages conversation and then turn the focus on the person to whom they are talking.
- Have a system for following up with contacts. Gracious people send a note or make a telephone call no later than 10 days after meeting a new contact, and anything they promised to follow up on will be done within that time as well.
- Are seen as "givers" in their community. Gracious networkers join organizations related to their business, and they get involved with the organization's activities. They are frequently seen at charity functions and are known for their ability to get things done.
- Network when things are going well, not only when they are not. Gracious individuals do not wait until a crisis to start networking; they share both good and bad times with their contacts.
- Listen. Gracious networkers concentrate exclusively on the individual with whom they are talking and do not allow themselves to be distracted by other people, for example, or by ambient noise in a room.
- Network with younger, less experienced individuals. Gracious networkers try to give as much as they get. They are not focused exclusively on networking up; they coach, counsel, and act as mentors for less experienced people.
- Leave conversations politely. Gracious networkers make polite excuses for leaving one conversation and joining another, rather than abruptly turning away and leaving the other individual to think that he or she was boring.
- Thank people. Gracious networkers are compulsive about giving thanks when they have received assistance, advice, or a business opportunity. Thus, they convey the message that they network not only for what they receive but for what they can give.

In addition to saying "thanks," it is important to pass on favors received through networking. The individual may not be able to pass on a favor to the individual from whom the initial favor was received, or pass on a favor of the same magnitude, or pass on a favor immediately. Regardless of these constraints, however, it is important to recognize and act on the reciprocity of networking. It is also effective to inform the individual granting the initial favor what has been done in exchange, such as: "I wanted to let you know that I was grateful for the opportunity to speak to the (name of group) for which you referred me; I have just referred Mary Smith for a similar opportunity."

Being gracious is an integral part of all interpersonal relationships. People who wish to be effective at networking must be able to socialize successfully with a variety of others.

Networking involves more than socializing skills, however. An individual who wishes to network effectively must have expertise in a field of practice, both to be credible and to be able to offer that expertise to those who may have need of it. Developing expertise in a particular field involves both educational and experiential credentials, and keeping up to date continuously (see chapter 3).

Making Conversation

Being able to converse with others is an essential networking skill. Many individuals are fearful of initiating a conversation with someone they do not know, particularly in a social situation, like a cocktail party, designed specifically for the purpose of networking. Gabor (1983) offers some helpful hints for would-be conversationalists:

- Be the first one to say "hello"; make eye contact with the individual and smile.
- Be confident and friendly, to put the other person at ease.
- Learn the person's name, and repeat it several times early in the conversation to help remember it.
- Offer a compliment or ask a question initially (preferably one that cannot be answered "yes" or "no").
- Focus opening remarks on the surroundings: the speakers, the meeting in general, the location, or the food.

Listen for cues to what the person wishes to discuss. Some people may have talked about work all day and prefer to discuss a social topic. In that case, pressing for details about the individual's occupation will bring the conversation to a rapid halt. Instead, follow up on what the person seems most interested in by asking additional questions.

Offering an opinion or information about oneself too soon may cause the conversation to falter and die. Encourage the other individual to talk until some common interest that can be pursued is uncovered. If one topic is exhausted, return to one that was raised earlier in the conversation. Use the person's name liberally during the discussion. Focus on the person instead of on the nurse consultant. Steer conversations away from controversial subjects, such as religion and politics; also, avoid gossip, complaints, or descriptions of unhappy events.

The nurse consultant's nonverbal communication during a conversation is as important as what is said, if not more so. Check body language frequently. Maintain eye contact, but do not stare; avoid the temptation to scan the room to see who else is there. Lean forward slightly, and nod to encourage the other person to keep talking. Stand with arms uncrossed. If holding a drink or plate, place the other hand in a pocket to avoid fidgeting and appearing bored with the conversation. Keep the hands away from the mouth: covering the mouth signals disapproval.

When the conversation appears to be finished, take leave gracefully. Avoid ending the conversation abruptly; rather, use the person's name and say how enjoyable the conversation has been. Recap briefly, particularly if any follow-up is planned, and then offer a noncommittal remark about needing to "circulate."

RoAne (1991) offers some helpful advice about handling cocktail parties and similar social situations with aplomb while accomplishing networking objectives:

- Look for someone who is alone, and start a conversation with him or her.
- Stand near the food, not the door. Individuals entering or leaving the room are not likely to want to be engaged in conversation, but those approaching the food will respond to comments about it.
- Play "host" by greeting others and making them feel welcome at the event.
- Plan good opening statements, although "Hi" or "Hello" often will suffice.
- Practice a self-introduction that will pique others' interest in further conversation.
- Approach groups of three or more to enter a conversation—never two individuals in an intense discussion.

Further, RoAne suggests that the individual attending a business cocktail party never forget his or her "business cards, . . . smile, nor . . . sense of humor" (p. 147). This excellent advice can be extended to all networking situations.

Managing Time for Networking

Most nurse consultants do not have a great deal of time to spend on networking, despite the obvious advantages. However, because of the value of networking to business, it is essential to carve out some time for it.

It may be necessary to eliminate some other activities to find the time for networking. Time management is a process to help eliminate activities that are least important so that time can be devoted to activities that are most important (see chapter 9).

To use the time management process, ask these questions, suggested by the authors of one of the leading texts on writing résumés (Krannich & Banis, 1982) in their discussion of career development and getting organized to search for a job:

- What do I want to accomplish?
- How am I organizing my activities to accomplish what I want?
- What results am I having in relation to what I want to accomplish?

Responses to these questions indicate the activities in which an individual is currently engaged.

Another way of assessing current activities is by keeping a daily log of activities in 15- to 30-minute increments. The log should be kept for at least a week, or preferably two weeks, to capture a typical range of activities. The log should include data describing the activity, its starting and ending times, who else was involved in it, who initiated it, and its end result. (This type of documentation of time spent in an activity is also useful in determining consultation fees; see chapter 5.)

Once it has been determined how the consultant's time is being spent, attention turns to managing time effectively so that time can be devoted to activities of most value, such as networking. Among the time management strategies that have been determined to be most helpful are the following (Puetz, 1983):

- Planning daily activities, both professional and personal
- Writing the daily plan as a "to do" list, including setting priorities for each activity and the anticipated time to be spent on the activity
- Reviewing the "to do" list the evening before
- Performing high-priority activities first, then less important activities
- Reviewing the list of activities frequently throughout the day to keep on track
- Noting in some fashion (e.g., checking off or striking through) which activities have been completed

In addition, time management experts recommend that an individual not attempt to do too much in one day; overscheduling leads to frustration. Other ways to maximize the time available to devote to a specific activity are to avoid interruptions; to delegate tasks that can easily be done by others; to organize work space for maximum efficiency; and, finally, to learn to say "no" to activities that are not contributing in some way to achievement of personal or professional goals. Eliminating nonessential activities from the nurse consultant's life may just free up time that can be devoted to networking.

Dressing for Success

Networking involves professional presence—making a good impression on others. Although the nurse consultant's appearance should not be the focus of networking efforts, first impressions are important (Bixler, 1992). Some fashion consultants describe the "power" of fashion, asserting that through fashion an individual expresses his or her professional as well as personal self. How an individual dresses reveals a lot about the individual (Fischer-Mirkin, 1995).

One key to dressing for success is not spending a great deal of money on clothes—money that could more profitably be used elsewhere. Some organized effort may result in a wardrobe that will meet the nurse consultant's need to look good at low cost.

Wardrobe.   Initial self-assessment is critical; the nurse consultant must review his or her current wardrobe for color, fit, and style. Clothes that do not fit or are hopelessly out of fashion should be discarded: give them away to friends, hold a garage sale, or donate them to a charity. (When items are donated, it is important to obtain a receipt for tax purposes.)

Items of clothing that have not been worn in the previous year also should be discarded, because it is highly unlikely that they will be worn in the future. Items of clothing that will be kept for their sentimental value should be carefully packed and stored in a location other than the closet in which an individual's "working wardrobe" is kept.

An existing wardrobe often can be extended if items are "mix and match." To ascertain which items go together, hang clothes in the closet by types: all jackets, all skirts, or trousers, and all blouses or shirts should be hung together. Thus, items that complement each other can be selected from each of the types of clothes in the closet.

It also may be helpful to hang ties or scarves that match jackets on the same hanger as the jacket. Jewelry for women, such as necklaces or bracelets, can be hung on these jacket hangers as well. Belts for both men and women can be hung on the jacket hangers. All this eliminates the need to search for complementary accessories when an outfit is selected.

Individuals in the nurse consultant's network can be asked to comment on various outfits. Spontaneous compliments also can provide clues to particularly flattering colors or styles.

An often overlooked resource is a "personal shopper." These individuals generally are found in large department stores and are employed by the department store. They advise buyers about clothing and accessory choices. The personal shopper will select an entire wardrobe based on the buyer's preferences (predetermined in an initial interview with the buyer). The buyer then tries on all the selections and purchases only those he or she prefers. There usually is no sales pressure, because pushing an unwanted item would result in the buyer's not returning. Personal shoppers offer candid feedback too; their livelihood depends on satisfied customers, so they do not want an individual to purchase something that does not look good on him or her. Most personal shoppers keep detailed files on their clients and often will call to suggest a "perfect" shirt to complement a man's suit, or a contrasting skirt that will increase the versatility of a woman's suit.

Although much of the advice offered by the fashion guru John Molloy is outdated (e.g., that women should wear only skirted suits in colors such as navy to work), some of his suggestions about shopping effectively are timeless. Molloy (1977) suggests several tips for buying clothes:

- Compare the price with anticipated use; items that will be used often can cost more than items worn only occasionally.
- Buy on sale, particularly at the end of a season.
- Be certain that markdowns are legitimate; knowing the merchandise in several stores and concentrating shopping in those stores will help avoid purchasing clothing that appears to be a bargain but is not.
- Buy clothes with a local merchant's label—the local merchant depends on repeat business, so clothing bearing a local merchant's label is more likely to be of high quality.
- Do not buy clothes with designer labels—clothing with designer labels tends to be high priced.
- Include cost of upkeep in the cost of the clothes—dry cleaning will add significantly to the cost of the clothing.
- Buy at discount stores or factory outlets, where designer-label clothing can often be found at a reduced price. Caution must be taken, however, to be sure that these items are not "irregulars" or "seconds."

Hairstyle. Because a person's hairstyle is an important part of professional presence, the nurse consultant's hairstyle should be flattering, easy to care for, and suitable for all occasions. The hairstyle should fit the person's face as well as his or her lifestyle.

To find the best hairstyle, make an appointment with a well-known and respected hair dresser. Recommendations from contacts are an excellent way to determine the name of such an hair stylist. Personal shoppers are good people to ask for recommendations, as are individuals whose hairstyles are particularly complimentary to them.

Ask the hair stylist for suggestions; some even have computer software programs that allow an individual to "try on" a variety of styles without ever touching the hair. Ask about upkeep of a preferred style: Color, tinting, and permanent waves add to the cost of maintaining a flattering look.

Makeup.   Makeup for women is an important part of their looks. Makeup must be applied appropriately for the activity in which the individual is engaged. Evening makeup is not appropriate for daytime wear, particularly in business situations.

Makeup consultation is available at most department stores. A personal shopper also can make recommendations about makeup—and often will suggest that makeup that will be worn with an outfit be applied before trying on the outfit. Regarding makeup in business situations, less is probably better.

Nails.   The recent trend for women to wear long artificial fingernails prompts some comments on the appropriate nail length for business. Nails should be kept short and clean. A light coat of polish is acceptable, but manicured nails that have been buffed to a shine are most attractive and suitable for business purposes. Artificial nails can be worn in the evenings and for other nonbusiness occasions.

Although wardrobe, makeup, and jewelry are not the entire focus of the nurse consultant's efforts as he or she plans and implements networking strategies, nonetheless they play an important part in preparation for successful networking. Meticulously groomed, individuals can feel confident in any and all networking situations that they are putting "their best foot forward," particularly when that foot is appropriately shod.

Networking at Meetings and Conferences

Tips to help overcome networking jitters when attending a professional meeting or conference (Smith, 1991) include preparing beforehand by contacting the sponsor's headquarters with a question about the program or a specific speaker. Find out if the individual to whom the nurse consultant is speaking will be at the meeting and if not, who will be the sponsor's representative. That way, there is someone to look for and meet on arrival at the conference location.

Introductions.   Set a reasonable goal for meeting people. It is overwhelming to think about meeting everyone at a conference, so choose a number and target networking efforts. Rehearse an introduction: It is deadly to provide too much information during an introduction, but it is equally conversation-stopping to just give a name and title. The opening statement should be brief but descriptive; "I'm Mary Smith, a consultant in pediatric rehabilitation. I help parents deal with a host of problems ranging from toilet training to adjusting to school after head injury."

Starting Conversations.   Plan at least a few questions to start a conversation: "How long have you been attending these meetings?" "What do you hope to learn here?" "How will you be able to use what you learn here in your business afterward?" (Note that these questions cannot be answered "yes" or "no"; thus they will not either stop the conversation or turn it into "20 Questions.")

Take advantage of every opportunity to talk with people—in the parking lot on arrival, in the registration line, in the hotel lobby, and in the elevator. These conversations do not have to be lengthy, but they provide an opportunity to meet some of the people who will be attending the conference over the next few days. These chance encounters can be turned into opportunities for the nurse consultant to greet these individuals by name every time he or she sees them. This simple technique will help the nurse consultant make an indelible impression—and be assured of being welcomed into a variety of groups throughout the meeting.

At all of the sessions during the meeting, sit strategically wherever there are empty seats nearby. Avoid joining tables that are nearly full; a conversation most likely is already in progress, and the newly arriving nurse consultant may be ignored. Joining someone who is sitting alone or with one or two others will guarantee a welcome.

Wearing Name Tags.   To facilitate introductions and conversations, it is important to wear at all times the name tag provided to conference attendees. Attach the name tag to the right side of the clothing so that an individual shaking hands can easily see the nurse consultant's name. Avoid covering the name tag with conference materials, even briefly. The lettering on the name tag should be large enough to read at a distance. If it is not, reverse the name tag and write the name and other identifying information in large block letters.

There almost certainly will be others at the conference who are uncomfortable too. Seek them out by scanning the room with a friendly smile. When someone makes eye contact in return and smiles, the nurse consultant has found a conversation partner. Focus efforts on people who are alone rather than trying to enter an existing group.

When meeting someone for the first time, remember that first impressions count. When attending a social event at an educational conference, for example, where potentially useful contacts are likely to be gathered, perform a quick once-over check before entering the room. In the rest room, check hair, teeth, and clothing. A man should straighten his tie; a woman should check her makeup and jewelry. Then, knowing that everything is in place makes meeting people easier.

Shaking Hands.   Shaking hands with individuals on meeting them is an American custom that should be followed. A simple handshake conveys a great deal about a person. Make eye contact with the individual and shake hands firmly; do not squeeze his or her hand and do not pump the clasped hands up and down. A woman should avoid a limp, fingers-only handshake; and a man should avoid covering the other person's hand— particularly a woman's—with both of his. Men and women both should shake hands on meeting someone; it is not necessary for a man to wait until the woman has extended her hand.

As the handshake is occurring, the nurse consultant offers an introduction. It is wise to use the other person's name first, such as, "Ann, I'm Mary Smith, a pediatric rehabilitation consultant." Repeat Ann's name again in the first few sentences; people like to hear their names, and repetition will help the nurse consultant remember the name.

Being Visible

Visibility is essential in networking. People must know who the nurse consultant is in order to be able to help him or her achieve his or her goals. Become visible in arenas where the contacts that can be of most assistance are also visible: in professional or community organizations, for example. Volunteer for office or offer to lead a project. Chair a committee or edit an organization's newsletter.

In a health care facility, volunteering to spearhead the United Way campaign can put an individual in the spotlight and provide unparalleled opportunities to interact with individuals from many different departments and areas of practice. Once the nurse consultant is successful at this effort, he or she may find many other opportunities coming along.

Take advantage of all of these—and any other—opportunities to speak, write for publication, be interviewed in the media, and work in volunteer and community organizations to expand the number of contacts with whom to network. Avoid the temptation to wait for opportunity to knock; the most successful people are those who make their own opportunities.

When Networking Does Not Work

Occasionally, an individual reports that "networking doesn't work for me!" On closer examination, however, it is apparent that the individual is not networking correctly.

For example, networking is not one-sided—it is a reciprocal arrangement where individuals "trade" favors. Networking must be perceived as valuable to both parties. Often, one individual may not be able to repay the other with a favor of the same magnitude, but it is important to acknowledge the assistance that has been received. Thank the person, publicly if possible. Follow up with a small gift, such as flowers or candy, or at the least a personal note in which the nurse consultant promises to pass on the assistance received.

Networking does not work if the nurse consultant abuses its purpose—for example, if the nurse consultant uses his or her position in a professional organization solely as a platform to promote his or her services. Another example is the nurse consultant who accepts referrals but never offers them to others.

Nor will networking work if the nurse consultant "uses" people, thinking only of what the contact can supply rather than what mutual benefits can accrue. Networking will not work if the nurse consultant fails to attend to the social rules, such as planning for more formal interactions with older individuals than with younger ones; obtaining introductions to these seniors through mutual acquaintances or membership in the same country club or social organization.

Networking *does* work if the nurse consultant practices skills in meeting people and talking with them and if the nurse consultant treats his or her contacts as he or she wishes to be treated. Networking with honesty and integrity as well as common courtesy will set the nurse consultant apart from many others and ensure his or her success in networking.

PUBLICITY CAMPAIGNS

To market services, the nurse consultant must "spread the word." Word of mouth is often the best advertising, but there are ways to implement a low-cost publicity campaign that will result in increased business (Smith, 1991). One of the most effective ways is to get press coverage of the nurse consultant's activities. If the nurse consultant's name appears in the local newspaper, for example, credibility with a potential client is enhanced, particularly if the news story emphasizes the nurse consultant's expertise.

Getting Media Coverage

It is not impossible to get one's name in print, but it is difficult. Following several steps will help (Burden, 1994).

Step 1: Send a Press Release.   First, the story the nurse consultant wants to get into the press must be newsworthy. To pique reporters' interest in the story, send out a press release. Write the press release using the five Ws of journalism: *who, what, where, when,* and *why.* Remember that the story must be interesting to the readers or listeners; a press release should not be advertising in disguise. Human interest stories sell well; if the nurse consultant has experienced a particularly satisfying encounter with a patient, for example, he or she may wish to publicize it. Also, consider stories on patients with rare or infrequent diseases, being careful not to violate confidentiality if others might recognize the patient from the story. A story on how the nurse consultant is setting up a consultation practice in a specific area of expertise may be newsworthy, if, for example, the nurse consultant's practice (prenatal care for low-income teens) coincides with something that is concurrently happening in the community (an increase in low-birthweight and failure-to-thrive infants). Such a story may receive a great deal of coverage. Sometimes a press release about a meeting at which the nurse consultant presented a paper or an article of the nurse consultant's that appeared in a nursing journal may result in an interview and a story about the nurse consultant and his or her business. Include a release date and a contact name and telephone number (Aronson & Spetner, 1993).

Step 2: Make a List of Media Contacts.   Developing media contacts is a networking activity in itself. Learn who's who in local radio, TV stations, and newspapers. If the nurse consultant's story is related to health care or business, target the media people who cover those areas. Know, too, who the audience is for the media outlet: Newspapers, for example, appeal to a different audience from television. Media outlets have demographics about their audience on file at their place of business. Make a visit to learn as much as possible, and try to meet the individual covering the nurse consultant's area of interest. The nurse consultant also may want to visit the local library to review media directories, particularly if she or he has a specific audience (e.g., African Americans or Hispanics) to reach. These directories often contain the names of editors and reporters for publications and radio and TV stations. Before sending a press release to a specific person, however, call to check that the person is still employed in the position.

Although it is possible to purchase targeted media lists from several of the publishers of these media directories, it may be best for the nurse consultant to create his or her own list, to be certain to market to the appropriate individuals and those with whom the nurse consultant has had some prior personal contact.

If the nurse consultant is fortunate enough to have someone from a public relations firm in his or her network, the nurse consultant can get a great deal of assistance. If not, do not hesitate to try to meet someone with expertise in public relations—at community functions, for example. The nurse consultant may be able to barter services in exchange for assistance with marketing his or her business.

Step 3: Follow Up.   Be sure to follow up once the press release has been sent. If the press release has been "mass mailed," the nurse consultant may not wish to call all the recipients; choose those from whom the nurse consultant has received a positive response previously. Ask the contact whether the press release was received and if the story is of interest. Then ask if further information is needed. If the individual sounds at all interested, try to make an appointment to discuss the story further. If the person is not interested, simply express thanks for his or her time and end the call.

Handling an Interview

In the event that the release paid off, and an interview is scheduled, the work actually begins. Tips for working effectively with the media include the following (Bixler, 1992):

1. Narrow the focus of the interview by deciding on the most interesting aspects of the services provided. Try to make only one or two points and make them well. Perhaps one important aspect of a nurse consultant's business may be the potential savings to employers when stress management techniques taught by the nurse consultant are used by employees. Another point may be that using these stress management techniques leads to satisfaction and lower turnover among employees. Weave these points into the interview.
2. If the interview is on television, ask the media contact if visual materials can be used. Then, bring photographs, slides, or items to demonstrate. This will provide variety in the presentation.
3. Plan clothing in advance. Blue is a good color to wear for a television interview. Avoid dark colors and white near the face (white appears harsh in the lights). Women should apply makeup that is a bit heavier than usual. When completely dressed for the interview, sit down in front of a full-length mirror, as the viewing audience will have that view as well. A suit jacket that fits perfectly when a man or woman is standing may bunch up unattractively when he or she is seated.
4. Express any concerns about the interview well before it begins. In the event that there is anything controversial about the topic under discussion, it is imperative that the interviewer is aware of it before the interview begins, in order for the interviewer and the guests not to be caught off guard. If there will be opposing viewpoints on the

topic, share with the interviewer what those viewpoints are likely to be and your position on them.

5. Take credit for accomplishments. Once an interview has been arranged, it is not the time to be modest and self-effacing. Interviewers and audiences want strong, self-confident individuals who can inform and entertain them.

6. Be open with the interviewer, but avoid revealing private information that can be taken out of context and prove detrimental later. Even with an assurance that the information will be "off the record," total candor generally is a mistake.

Capitalize on the exposure created by the interview by sending an announcement of the interview to the local newspaper and to other media outlets previously targeted. Often a radio station will follow up on a television interview, judging the topic "newsworthy" if it has been aired, or a television station will follow up on a radio interview.

NETWORKING GROUPS

Networking occurs informally, but there are groups organized for the specific purpose of networking. The National Association of Female Executives (NAFE), for example, has established local networking groups in areas around the country. NAFE also conducts networking meetings for its members. For information about NAFE, see the Appendix.

Other organizations with which the nurse consultant may wish to network include the National Nurses in Business Association, the National Association of Women Business Owners, and others. Telephone listings for these groups are found in the Yellow Pages; or they can be contacted though listings of their meetings in the business section of local newspapers.

Opportunities for networking also may be found in membership directories of professional societies. Some publications, such as the *American Journal of Nursing*, provide readers with a directory of specialty nursing organizations, state nurses associations, and state boards of nursing annually. JONA publishes a "Directory of Nursing Consultants" in which individuals with whom the nurse consultant may wish to network are listed.

SUMMARY

Networking is an easy and effective tool for nurse consultants. Although it takes time to organize networking efforts and network effectively, that time generally is well spent. The payoffs from networking should not be underestimated. Meeting, keeping, and using contacts to accomplish professional goals is a well-known strategy for career success: "It's not *what* you know, but *who* you know!"

Networking involves being prepared, being confident, looking good, making conversation, and being gracious. Following the rules of networking is a key to success. Networking has worked for men for ages and is working now for women as well.

Although there are risks involved in networking—meeting people, knowing what to say, being certain to follow up and keep in touch—the ultimate benefits of networking activities provide convincing evidence that networking is crucial to professional success.

REFERENCES

Aronson, M., & Spetner, D. (1993). *Public relations writer's handbook.* Lexington, MA: Lexington.

Bixler, S. (1992). *Professional presence.* New York: Perigree.

Burden, D. (1994, July/August). Do-it-yourself publicity. *Executive Female,* pp. 71–72.

Deep, S., & Sussman, L. (1990). *Smart moves.* Reading, MA: Addison-Wesley.

Fischer-Mirkin, T. (1995). *Dress code.* New York: Clarkson Potter.

Fisher, D., & Vilas, S. (1992). *Power networking* (2nd ed.). Austin, TX: Mountain-Harbour.

Gabor, D. (1983). *How to start a conversation and make friends.* New York: Simon & Schuster.

Hauter, J. (1993). *The smart woman's guide to career success.* Hawthorne, NJ: Career Press.

Kelly, L. Y., & Joel, L. A. (1995). *Dimensions of professional nursing* (7th ed.). New York: McGraw-Hill.

Krannich, R. L., & Banis, W. J. (1982). *High impact resumes and letters.* Chesapeake, VA: Progressive Concepts.

Malloy, J. T. (1977). The woman's dress for success book. New York: Warner.

Puetz, B. E. (1983). *Networking for nurses.* Rockville, MD: Aspen.

Puetz, B. E. (1991). Networking: Making it work for you. *Health Care Trends and Transitions, 3,* 20–24.

Puetz, B. E. (1993). Networking. In D. J. Mason, S. W. Talbott, & J. K. Leavitt (Eds.), *Policy and politics for nurses* (2nd ed., pp. 179–183). Philadelphia: W. B. Saunders.

RoAne, S. (1991). *How to work a room.* New York: Warner.

Smith, J. (1991). *The publicity kit.* New York: John Wiley & Sons.

Smith, L. (1991, January/February). Solo networking. *Executive Female,* p. 49.

Smith, L. (1993, January/February). Do the right people know you? *Executive Female,* p. 56.

Smith, L. (1995, September/October). Never fail to be gracious. *Executive Female,* p. 74.

Stern, B. B. (1981). *Is networking for you?* Englewood Cliffs, NJ: Prentice-Hall.

Welch, M. S. (1980). *Networking.* New York: Harcourt Brace Jovanovich.

Zagury, C. S. (1993). *Nurse entrepreneur.* Long Branch, NJ: Vista.

8

Ethical and Legal Considerations in Consulting

Ethics are virtues, values, or views people possess about what is good or bad, right or wrong. Ethics are often spoken of in terms of morality or acceptable behavior. Churchill (1977) suggests that "Morality is generally defined as behavior according to custom or tradition. Ethics, by contrast, is the free, rational assessment of courses of action in relation to precepts, rules, conduct. . . . To be ethical a person must take the additional step of exercising critical, rational judgment in his decisions" (p. 873). Ethical persons accept accountability and responsibility for their actions and behaviors and predicate those actions and behaviors on tenets gained from their upbringing, background, and education, and the creeds of the discipline or group with which they associate or to which they belong.

ETHICAL ASPECTS OF CONSULTATION

Codes of Ethics

Acceptable ways to behave or deal with ethical questions are often guided by codes of conduct or behavior. For example, the Boy Scout pledge, the Nightingale pledge, and the Hippocratic oath are all guides to actions or behavior.

In nursing, the *Code for Nurses with Interpretative Statements* (American Nurses Association, 1976), first crafted in 1926, is the doctrine that governs the practice and behavior of the nurse. The interpretive statements explain the planks of the code and suggest ways the nurse can carry out and measure up to the code. Although the "Code for Nurses" (see Table 8.1) was most likely not written with the nurse consultant in mind, several of the 11 planks of the code contain guidance for the nurse consultant.

For example, plank 2 speaks to the need for the nurse to guard clients' confidences. Certainly, the nurse consultant has an obligation to hold in confidence proprietary information given by the client and must guard against releasing information without the client's permission. Information given to the consultant in confidence during the data-gathering stage of the consultation must be held in secret as well.

Another example is plank 5, about maintaining competence in nursing. The consultant must maintain competence in a specialty or area of expertise and not try to provide advice beyond that competence. Plank 5 augurs for continual learning and updating one's knowledge base.

Plank 7 urges the nurse to contribute to the body of knowledge of the profession on an ongoing basis. Those nurses who are serving as consultants or intrapreneurs within a health care institution are good examples of taking nursing knowledge and contributing it to nurse colleagues, thereby enhancing the knowledge of others.

Interestingly, plank 6 actually mentions consultation. Although plank 6 refers to the nurse seeking consultation, it is equally applicable to the nurse consultant giving consultation. Plank 6 states, "The nurse exercises informed judgment and uses individual competence and qualifications as criteria in seeking consultation, accepting responsibilities, and delegating nursing activities to others" (American Nurses Association, 1976). The use of judgment and individual competence is certainly critical in fulfilling the role of consultant, and having the qualifications to consult is equally important. As noted earlier, accepting responsibility is one of the hallmarks of the ethical person.

A word about delegation is in order here. From time to time, the consultant may need to engage a helper or another consultant to work on a project or a part of a consulting assignment. The consultant must be certain that any assistant is capable and qualified to do the job; that the requirements of the job including time lines and due dates are explained clearly; and that the person to whom the work is assigned has the tools and training to do the job. The delegating consultant must be careful to follow up on the work delegated and be sure the job is done competently, correctly, and on time.

As noted in chapter 1, the Institute of Management Consultants (IMC) has approved a "Code of Ethics" for those in management consulting (see Table 8.2) that addresses work with clients and the behavior of the consultant. The IMC code refers to confidentiality, as does the code for nurses. The IMC code also refers to the competence of the practicing consultant, much as the code for nurses mentions the competence of the practicing nurse. Also, the code for nurses addresses the nursing profession's obligation

TABLE 8.1   American Nurses Association Code for Nurses

Preamble

The Code for Nurses is based on belief about the nature of individuals, nursing, health and society. Recipients and providers of nursing services are viewed as individuals and groups who possess basic rights and responsibilities, and whose values and circumstances command respect at all times. Nursing encompasses the promotion and restoration of health, the prevention of illness, and the alleviation of suffering. The statements of the Code and their interpretation provide guidance for conduct and relationships in carrying out nursing responsibilities consistent with the ethical obligations of the profession and quality in nursing care.

1. The nurse provides services with respect for human dignity and the uniqueness of the client unrestricted by considerations of social or economic status, personal attributes, or the nature of health problems.
2. The nurse safeguards the client's right to privacy by judiciously protecting information of a confidential nature.
3. The nurse acts to safeguard the client and the public when health care and safety are affected by the incompetent, unethical, or illegal practice of any person.
4. The nurse assumes responsibility and accountability for individual nursing judgments and actions.
5. The nurse maintains competence in nursing.
6. The nurse exercises informed judgment and uses individual competence and qualifications as criteria in seeking consultation, accepting responsibilities, and delegating nursing activities to others.
7. The nurse participates in activities that contribute to the ongoing development of the profession's body of knowledge.
8. The nurse participates in the profession's efforts to implement and improve standards of nursing.
9. The nurse participates in the profession's efforts to establish and maintain conditions of employment conducive to high quality nursing care.
10. The nurse participates in the profession's effort to protect the public from misinformation and misrepresentation and to maintain the integrity of nursing.
11. The nurse collaborates with members of the health professions and other citizens in promoting community and national efforts to meet the health needs of the public.

Source: Code for Nurses with Interpretive Statements. Reprinted with permission of the American Nurses Association.

TABLE 8.2   Code of Ethics

CODE OF ETHICS

Clients

1. We will serve our clients with integrity, competence, and objectivity.

2. We will keep client information and records of client engagements confidential and will use proprietary client information only with the client's permission.

3. We will not take advantage of confidential client information for ourselves or our firms.

4. We will not allow conflicts of interest which provide a competitive advantage to one client through our use of confidential information from another client who is a direct competitor without that competitor's permission.

Engagements

5. We will accept only engagements for which we are qualified by our experience and competence.

6. We will assign staff to client engagements in accord with their experience, knowledge, and expertise.

7. We will immediately acknowledge any influences on our objectivity to our clients and will offer to withdraw from a consulting engagement when our objectivity or integrity may be impaired.

Fees

8. We will agree independently and in advance on the basis for our fees and expenses and will charge fees and expenses that are reasonable, legitimate, and commensurate with the services we deliver and the responsibility we accept.

9. We will disclose to our clients in advance any fees or commissions that we will receive for equipment, supplies or services we recommend to our clients.

Profession

10. We will respect the intellectual property rights of our clients, other consulting firms, and sole practitioners and will not use proprietary information or methodologies without permission.

11. We will not advertise our services in a deceptive manner and will not misrepresent the consulting profession, consulting firms, or sole practitioners.

12. We will report violations of this Code of Ethics.

The Council of Consulting Organizations, Inc. Board of Directors approved this Code of Ethics on January 8, 1991.
The Institute of Management Consultants (IMC) is a division of the Council of Consulting Organizations. Inc.

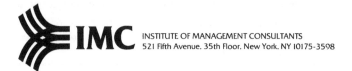 IMC   INSTITUTE OF MANAGEMENT CONSULTANTS
521 Fifth Avenue. 35th Floor. New York. NY 10175-3598

Reprinted with permission of the Institute of Management Consultants.

to protect the public from misinformation and misrepresentation, and the code of ethics for management consultants addresses the consulting profession's obligation not to engage in deceptive advertising or misrepresentation.

Although such codes are important tools for the nurse consultant, people in today's society are quite cynical about the products and services of others, including credos or rules of behavior articulated by professional groups. Indeed, in some circles, *consultant* is a dirty word and consultants may occasionally experience a hostile, unfriendly environment and attitude. Such cynicism can best be met by a reputation that is impeccable; a work product that is of high quality; and competency, honesty, and fairness in all dealings. In fact, the consultant's reputation is probably his or her most important asset.

Ethical Conduct

Holtz (1993) offers guidance on the matter of ethical conduct. This guidance applies to internal and external nurse consultants. Holtz suggests consideration of the following ethical standards. Item 5 needs no embellishment; the rest are discussed briefly below.

1. Deliver what you promise.
2. Do not withhold facts or embellish the truth to purposefully mislead the client.
3. Respect confidences.
4. Honestly account for time spent. Be honest in all dealings with clients and prospective clients.
5. Do not "bad mouth" other consultants.
6. Engage in dignified, professional conduct—always.
7. Deal with others, such as vendors and suppliers, as you would with clients.

Promises. A consultant's word is golden. A pledge of competency in undertaking an assignment agreed on; a warranty for finishing work in a manner and time line consented to; and a guarantee of a product for a specified price must be honored. In other words, the consultant must do what he or she says he or she will do. To do otherwise is unethical.

Facts. A misstatement or manipulation of facts or words to "put a good face" on bad news or to lead a client in a direction that may be questionable is just plain wrong. Do not do it.

Confidences. Keeping clients' confidences is one of the major rules of the nursing and consulting professions. To divulge a confidence not only is unethical but breaks the tenets and traditions of the professions. Betrayal of clients' confidences not only besmirches the nurse consultant but also reflects on all who might provide consulting services and helps perpetuate public cynicism about consultants.

Honesty.   A practice of being honest in all dealings with clients is the best policy. Telling the truth, no matter how painful, is the best practice for the nurse consultant to follow. From time to time, a client will ask for facts to be altered or distorted. Both the ANA "Code for Nurses" and the IMC "Code of Ethics" address the obligation of the professional to avoid misrepresentation. The issue of misrepresentation of information will be addressed later in this chapter, under the heading "Shades of Gray."

Conduct.   The manner in which the nurse consultant conducts himself or herself speaks volumes. Off-color language, gossiping, jokes that poke fun at groups of people, inappropriate or inadequate dress, an office in disarray, or reports filled with typographical errors or coffee stains are not befitting of a nurse consultant or an ethical approach to consulting practice. Dignified behavior, appropriate to the setting and circumstances, mirrors the consultant's judgmental abilities and speaks volumes about the consultant's work products. The consultant's demeanor and deportment are also a marketing tool—one that can be effective in attracting clients or sending clients to another consultant.

Dealings.   Plank 1 of the "Code for Nurses" calls on the nurse to provide services with respect for human dignity and the uniqueness of the client irrespective of health or economic or social status. Such respect should be accorded by the nurse consultant to clients, clients' employees, colleagues, and all with whom consultant does business. How the nurse consultant treats others will be known in the marketplace and can either make or break a consulting practice.

Ethics and the Law

Ethics are not synonymous with law or obeying the law but are principles a step above or beyond what is required by law. In that respect, ethics involves obedience to the unenforceable (Guttenberg, 1995). There is no court of law to which one can take a claim of unethical behavior. Although there are trade and professional associations that set forth codes of ethics, there is often little opportunity to enforce those codes beyond revoking membership privileges in the association. In many instances, those acting unethically do not belong to a trade or professional organization and are therefore beyond the reach of the association. The consultant who acts unethically is most likely to be censored in the marketplace by a tarnished reputation and declining business.

Ethical values and principles should be included in every consultant's tool kit. Ethical values and principles are embodied in many documents, codes, organization position statements, standards, and rules of conduct. Consultants' organizations, like most trade and professional associations and even many businesses, have guidelines for acceptable practices or behaviors. Whether the ten commandments, the golden rule, a professional code of ethics, or the nurse consultant's personal values and principles, it is good to have a reference point when a situation arises that may be potentially improper. Whether the reference point is a formally written code of conduct or a "gut feeling," the consultant should decide what is ethical and what is not and practice accordingly.

Ethics and the Consultation Process

Consultation is an activity built on trust between the client and consultant. The ethical behaviors of both influence the process and outcome of the consultation. Ethical issues can arise at any point during the consultation process. How to respond to an ethical predicament is in many respects a judgment call. The wise nurse consultant thinks about the likelihood of ethical issues and prepares to respond to them before the situation occurs. Ulschak and SnowAntle (1990) describe ethical problems that can arise in the following stages of the consultation process:

1. Contractual
2. Data collection
3. Data presentation
4. Action plan
5. Evaluation

Following is a brief discussion of each of these stages of the consultation process and the ethical issues that may occur at each stage. To these five stages the authors have added a sixth:

6. Billing

Contractual. In this phase of the consultation process, the consultant reaches agreement with the client about the scope of the project; what is to be done, by whom, and when; the roles of the consultant and the client; and the fee to be paid for the project. During this phase, one ethical issue that may arise, related to the work to be done, may result from the consultant's not having the skills to perform satisfactorily. What can be done?

The consultant may choose to accept the project, despite not knowing if he or she is capable of completing it; or the consultant may refer the project to another consultant who does have the necessary skills. It is essential that the client be informed if the consultant has not previously worked with a project of this nature; then, together, they can decide how to proceed.

An even more delicate example is the situation in which the consultant bids on a proposal and the contract is awarded to a competitor who the consultant knows does not have skills or expertise to do the job or who has completed a similar project for another client in a very unsatisfactory manner. What can be done? The nurse consultant might be tempted to report the other consultant to the appropriate professional association, or to tell the client. Although both are possible options, the inherent danger is the potential that the nurse consultant does not have all the facts surrounding the situation and that he or she might be viewed as a teller of tales that are not true or the carrier of a story that is already known. For example, the competitor might have reported to the client the misadventures with another client, or the competitor might be bringing an associate to the assignment who does have the relevant skills or expertise. Another alternative is for the nurse consultant to speak to the competitor and express questions or concerns. Although this might be perceived by the competitor as inappropriate, unbecoming, or a fear of competition and little might be determined, it is one way in which the nurse consultant can raise concerns related to practice. More often than not, the consultant who has concerns about a competitor will likely do nothing, relying on the marketplace to weed out the incompetent and unethical.

Another ethical issue at the contractual stage of the consultation process relates to the relationship between client and consultant. Perhaps the client intends to use the findings of the project in ways with which the consultant disagrees. For example, the client decides to offer a training course to nurses in the community in order to raise money when the client knows that the training, already pilot tested in the clients' setting, has a negligible impact on practice or patient outcomes. A possible action for the consultant in this instance is to inform the client of the value conflict and if no resolution can be achieved, to decline the consultation.

Other ethical problems that may emerge during the contractual stage of the consultation process involve the consultant's agreeing to objectives that will be impossible to achieve in the time frame allocated to the project. Sometimes this unfortunate circumstance occurs because the consultant is eager to have the project for the income it will bring to the business, and so thinks it would be better to accept the contract and worry about what has to be done later rather than risk losing the business by telling the client the expectations are unrealistic. Withholding information about unreasonable expectations is unethical and damaging to the client-consultant relationship. If the assignment cannot be completed as promised or if the job is completed and the work is shoddy, the consultant's reputation, credibility, and ethics are on the line. At the time of the writing of this book, one of the authors responded to a client's request for consultation, noting that the client's time line could not be met by the consultant but that the work could be completed 2 weeks after the date proposed by the client. The client could not or would not wait for the additional 2 weeks, and the consultant "lost" the business. How easy it would have been to have agreed to complete the assignment by the date required and either rushed the job or missed the date.

Data Collection. During this phase of consulting work, the consultant collects information, through a variety of methods, about the problem to be solved. In this stage, decisions also are made about who will provide the information and how the data will be collected.

Ethical dilemmas that may arise during this stage involve the collection of unnecessary data, which wastes precious resources, such as time. The consultant may conduct interviews with a variety of individuals within the institution, not all of whom are essential to collect the needed information. This scenario may occur because the consultant has not performed this type of project previously and, therefore, is uncertain how to do it. Thus, in addition to unwise expenditure of the consultant's time, the organization is charged for the time of the individuals involved in the interviews for no appreciable purpose. On the other hand, the consultant might run out of time to collect data that had been promised but prepares the report in such a way as to imply that the data were collected, when that was not the case. Either practice is dishonest and unethical.

Another potential ethical plight is not sharing limitations related to data collection with the client at the outset of the consultation. The consultant also could withhold information that may not address the client's concerns, or data that will not please the client. All of these are instances of unethical practice on the part of the consultant.

Data Presentation. The data-presentation stage of the consultation process is described by Ulschak and SnowAntle (1990) as the period during which the consultant analyzes the data that have been collected and presents them to the client. During this stage, the consultant may face an ethical predicament regarding how to present the data; perhaps the wrong data were gathered because of the consultant's inexperience, or the consultant does not know how to present the data, or the consultant's own bias colors the reporting of the data. Perhaps the consultant withholds negative data that may affect the decisions made about the project by the client, or the consultant fears that presentation of negative data might result in no future business from the client. In each of these situations, the consultant is acting unethically by misrepresentation or withholding necessary information from the client.

Action Plan.   In this stage of the consultation process, the consultant and client make decisions about what needs to be done, by whom, and under what conditions to accomplish the objectives of and recommendations emanating from the project. During this phase, ethical issues arise if the previous steps have not been performed according to ethical principles. If any information has been withheld or misrepresented for fear of alienating the client, or if the information is erroneous, the resulting action plan will not be on target. The consequences for the client are legion and could include faulty business decisions, causing loss of many dollars; injury to patients; poor employee relations; or a sullied reputation in the marketplace. The consequences for the consultant should be obvious; they include a clouded reputation and even potential legal action.

Evaluation.   During the evaluation phase of the consultation process, the client and consultant review the effectiveness of the consultation: what was accomplished versus what was supposed to be accomplished. Either the consultation was a success, or it was not. If not, then the client needs to decide whether to continue to pursue the project and attempt to complete it, or discontinue further efforts. The consultant needs to determine whether he or she performed to the best of his or her ability. If the consultant made errors or did not do a good job, then the consultant must determine whether to do the work over, refund or reduce the fee or part of the fee, or provide another avenue for the client to accomplish the job. An ethical issue can occur during this phase if the client does not have sufficient information to make a decision about the success of the project because the information was withheld by the consultant.

Billing.   When the consultation ends, there is the matter of billing. Although Ulschak and SnowAntle (1990) do not list billing as a specific stage of the consulting process, the authors believe it is an important part of the consulting process and one that can tempt the consultant to act unethically.

Fees should be agreed to during the contractual stage of the consultation. Although billing a client for work done and expenses incurred seems like a straightforward matter, the consultant may have expended more time completing an assignment than anticipated and thus may pad an invoice for direct expenses to attempt to obtain payment for some of the hours that could not be billed. Another consultant may discover business expenses that are unexpected and thus may be tempted to pad the expense line on several assignments to replace losses and increase earnings.

Consultants must adhere to fee schedules and must be honest in recovering expenses. Should an assignment take more time than planned for when the fee was agreed to, the consultant has several options:

1. Call the additional time to the client's attention and try to negotiate an additional fee. This is best done as soon as the consultant realizes that the time allotted for the work will be exceeded.
2. Call the additional work to the client's attention, pointing out that no extra fee will be charged and that the consultant looks forward to working with the client on a future assignment.
3. Say nothing, absorb the loss, and learn from the experience when calculating fees for future assignments.

In the survey of nurse consultants conducted by the authors in mid-1995, of those responding to a question about costs running over the contract for the consultation, half of respondents ($n = 114$, 50%) absorb cost overruns, and 31% ($n = 114$) renegotiate the fee structure and work output. Of those responding to a question about costs running below projections, 49% ($n = 99$) report doing nothing, 23% ($n = 99$) report renegotiating fee structure and output, and 20% ($n = 99$) report either negotiating a lower fee structure or negotiating an increase in work output.

From time to time, a client will ask for more work to be done as a part of a consultation project, such as additional data gathering or interviews with a larger number of people. When the client asks for additional work to be done, the consultant should respond with information about an increase in charges, given the work requested. It may be appropriate to amend the client-consultant contract. The client's bill should not automatically include a fee increase at the end of the assignment unless the client has agreed to the additional charges.

An invoice for reimbursement of expenses should be accompanied by an itemized list of expenditures accompanied by all applicable receipts. From time to time, out-of-pocket expenses, such as a pay telephone call, do not result in having a receipt to provide the client. In that case, adequate explanation of the expense (such as the purpose of the call and the party called) should satisfy the client as to the legitimacy of the expenditure.

Other Ethical Issues

Another ethical plight occurs when the consultant shares data inappropriately with others. For example, the consultant divulges a new product in development, a pricing scheme, or information about personnel to a prospective client. Such an event is likely to occur when the consultant is bidding on a similar project, and in an effort to obtain the contract, tells what he or she knows about another client in an effort to influence receipt of new business.

Consultants can be confronted with a myriad of indecorous situations. A consultant may uncover unlawful behavior such as theft of drugs, falsification of records, or tax fraud; or a consultant may be asked to change recommendations in a report to present a more favorable picture of an organization or its CEO.

In every instance of illegal or unlawful behavior uncovered in an organization, the exploit should be brought to the attention of the CEO for immediate action. Although it is tempting to advise immediate reporting of the matter to the authorities, there is no set rule that covers every situation. If the CEO rectifies the situation and brings the matter to the attention of the proper authorities, the matter may be settled as far as the consultant is concerned. If the CEO takes no action, the consultant is best advised to contact legal counsel, explain the situation, present the agreement with the client, and act accordingly. In a rare situation, the uncovering of a heinous crime or illegal act should be reported to the authorities without delay. Perhaps the best guidance in such a situation is immediate consultation with the consultant's own attorney.

If the illegal acts uncovered have been perpetrated by the CEO, the consultant should consult with legal counsel to determine the most appropriate action. The consultant should probably call the matter to the attention of the CEO, presenting any evidence that exists. The specter of confronting a CEO with evidence of criminal behavior is daunting at best. Depending on the circumstances, the consultant may wish to have another individual, such as a business partner, along at such a meeting for support and security. Reporting the discovery to the CEO's supervisor—for example, a board of trustees—and to the authorities should be handled in consultation with the consultant's legal counsel and must be based on hard evidence, not on hearsay or circumstantial signs or symptoms.

Most people know when an act violates their acceptable ethical principles and values. If the nurse consultant is wondering whether or not a matter or practice is ethical, or has a troubled conscience, it is likely that his or her principles and values may be about to be violated.

Weiss (1992) urges attention to the following guidelines to determine if the consultant is doing the right thing:

1. Is the activity under consideration one that will improve the client's condition or the consultant's?
2. Is the action something the consultant is comfortable explaining to the client?
3. Is the activity something the consultant can be proud of and would publicize readily?

4. Could harm occur to anyone without an opportunity for that person to respond?
5. Is the approach one to which the consultant would willingly submit?

These same questions are good ones for the consultant to ask when confronting behavior on the part of a client that does not seem quite right, when deciding what advice to give, or when deciding whether or not to take on a client. In the survey of nurse consultants conducted by the authors in mid-1995, 34% (34 of 99) of those responding to a question related to confronting a potentially unethical situation reported withdrawing from the situation; 47% (47 of 99) reported attempting to change the situation while continuing with the contract.

Examples: Shades of Gray

Examples of situations consultants might encounter that call for ethical judgments follow. Cohen (1991) reports that many of the situations can be predicted by the consultant.

"Don't Tell The Boss."   Once in a while, a consultant will run across a client who wants to spare the boss bad news or information that does not reflect favorably on an employee or the organization. The consultant is asked to cushion the presentation of information or to eliminate information from a report—such a request is usually followed by assurances that the matter will be brought to the boss's attention in another way.

Although a consultant's findings can be reported in such a way as to not be hurtful, deliberately withholding information is not appropriate or ethical. However, some consultants contend that information not having a direct bearing on the consulting assignment or direct relevance to the findings and recommendations can be withheld and not compromise the consultant or the client.

Cohen (1991) reports that some clients want the consultant to lie to the boss. Cohen notes that some consultants will go along with a little "white lie," but others refuse to lie no matter the circumstances. The authors advise honest and full disclosure as the best policy.

"You Can't Say That In Your Report."   This is akin to "Don't tell the boss." Be prudent in responding to such a request. The consultant might say something in a different way or consider giving the information orally. Information that is critical to the findings and recommendations of the consultant should not be withheld; this is dishonest and not only can injure the credibility of the consultant but can also result in business decisions that are injurious to the client.

"Why Not Fudge the Data? No One Will Get Hurt."   There are ample reports in the media, business, and research of falsification, misstatement, or misinterpretation of data. If the nurse consultant developed the data, the nurse consultant should be clear and accurate in reporting the findings. If the consultant is using other data sources, a check should be made to ensure that the data sources are reliable, and the consultant should *always* give credit or attribution to the sources used.

"Can You Get Me a Job at the XYZ Company?"   The successful consultant has a lot of contacts. Thus, it is natural for colleagues and clients or clients' workers to ask for help in getting a job, especially in an environment plagued by job uncertainty. The consultant may also have an entrée into a company that a client has always wanted to work for. A request for help in getting a client or a client's employee a job merits caution. Except in rare circumstances, the nurse consultant should not be the link between a client's employees and a prospective employer. Should the nurse consultant be viewed as robbing a client of valued employees, the nurse consultant is likely not to be invited back and may get a reputation of luring employees away from clients.

Cohen (1991) suggests that a client is no longer a client after 5 years pass with no new assignments. Cohen reports that headhunters regard clientele as lasting no longer than 3 years. The nurse consultant must weigh and measure helping clients or clients' employees get a job with another company. There is no one right answer for every situation.

"Here's What We Want You to Say in the Report."   This statement is often heard when an organization knows what it wants to do about a matter but an independent third-party verification is needed. The verification might be requested by a supervisor, could be sought to give validity to an opinion or an undertaking, or might be obtained as a way to justify an action. An outsider's view can also be used to persuade doubters or "those on the fence" internally or externally.

Although giving an organization the desired consultation outcome might be an easy way to earn money, the consultant must not be lulled into supporting findings and recommendations that are a sham or do not result from the consultant's own observations, findings, or knowledge base. One example comes from the author's recent experience with a state-based health care organization. The organization's board engaged the author to do a feasibility study related to entering a new business venture. The group asked the consultant to do the study under the assumption that the new business venture was desirable and feasible. The consultant's findings proved that the endeavor was not a good idea and that another approach was warranted. The consultant reported these findings and recommended that the health care organization take a different approach. Although a few members of the organization's board were disturbed that the consultant did not tell them what they expected and wanted to hear, the organization's CEO and president were impressed that the consultant adhered to the findings and crafted recommendations accordingly rather than give the group what they wanted to hear.

Cohen (1991) suggests that the consultant think about the alternatives for responding to such a request early in a consulting career, because the situation will arise sooner or later. Cohen also advises that there is no one right answer.

"What Did You Find Out When Consulting for the ABC Firm?" A consultant may work for competitors and be asked by one to reveal information about the other. Divulging proprietary information is unethical and may be illegal. Often a client will ask for assurances of confidentiality from the consultant, to be written into the consulting agreement. The wise consultant will provide a confidentiality statement in any proposal or agreement for consulting services.

On the rare occasion that information from a rival organization might be appropriate to the consultant's work, permission to divulge the information should always be obtained prior to doing so. If the permission cannot be obtained, do not divulge the information. One possible option for handling such a situation is to suggest that company X might have information that would be of help or interest to company Y and that company Y might want to consult company X. Care must be used in exercising this option so as not to divulge clients' confidences.

Much of what a consultant brings to an assignment is reputation. A consultant makes a living on reputation. A reputation marred by unethical behavior or practices can deprive the consultant of business. Behavior by a consultant that is clearly unethical includes falsifying credentials; padding invoices; borrowing others' ideas and failing to give credit for them; divulging confidences when the consultant has agreed to keep something confidential; and stretching or falsifying data.

LEGAL ASPECTS OF CONSULTATION

Many aspects of the consulting business require knowledge of certain legal principles; awareness of potential risk in decision making; familiarity with laws, rules, or regulations related to structuring a consulting business; and information about how certain laws or regulations might apply to a client and the advice the consultant might give a client. In no way should the information in this chapter be construed as legal advice. The information is provided to sensitize the reader to potential issues and to the need for competent legal counsel in those situations where counsel is needed. In addition, the Small Business Administration (SBA) and small-business development offices located at many colleges and universities across the country can often answer some of the basic legal questions regarding starting a business, business planning, business structure, and so forth.

Selecting Legal Counsel

Although it might be tempting to turn to a lawyer friend or acquaintance or the lawyer who wrote the nurse consultant's will or represented the consultant in divorce proceedings, do not take this easy route. Lawyers specialize in various aspects of the law (as nurses specialize in various aspects of nursing), and some are better than others. In fact, a good way to go about selecting legal counsel is to use the strategies clients use when selecting a nurse consultant.

Fallek (1991) advises talking to people who own other small businesses in the neighborhood or community to determine the lawyer or law firm with which they do business. Ask how satisfied the small-business owner is with the service provided; for example, how promptly the attorney returns calls. Ask about the types of situations in which the owner has used counsel and whether or not the representation was perceived as adequate. Also, inquire about fees. Ask, "What were the fees?" If the nurse consultant is not comfortable asking for this information directly or the owner is unwilling to share the specific fees, ask:

> "What is your perception of the attorney's fees?"
> "Did the attorney charge for every telephone call made to the law office?"
> "Did the attorney take the time to get to know the business of the client and visit the business site?"

Identify three to five lawyers to interview. When contacting an attorney, ask for an appointment to interview the potential counsel at no cost. If this opportunity is denied, the nurse consultant does not want to work with this lawyer and should try another. Prepare for the appointment in advance. Go the public library and look the attorney up in one of the references available. A good reference is *Martindale-Hubbell Law Directory* (1995). This reference, published for each state, will give the nurse consultant information about the attorney's education, type of practice, location, and affiliation with a firm; the longevity of the firm; the firm's major clients; and the bar or bars to which the attorney has been admitted. The nurse consultant can call the bar association and ask if the lawyer is in good standing. The American Association of Nurse Attorneys might also provide information and can be contacted by writing to 3525 Ellicott Mills Drive, Suite N, Ellicott City, MD 21043-4547, or telephoning 410-418-4800.

Prepare a list of questions for the interview. They might include the following:

1. The attorney's major area or areas of practice and expertise.
2. The attorney's familiarity with the consultant's line of business.
3. List of references of current clients that counsel represents who are in a line of business similar to the consultant's. (Check some of these references, but also check references of clients not on the reference list.)
4. Fee schedule and how the fee schedule is determined. Lawyers often use the same fee scheme as consultants (i.e., hourly or by assignment). Lawyers may also prefer a contingency fee; that is, a percentage of an amount obtained through settlement of litigation. Be sure to ask about fees and about charges for telephone calls. When the consultant is first starting out, he or she may check with counsel more frequently. Thus, the consultant should not be surprised by the bill. And, like the consultant, the lawyer will usually charge the customer for any out-of-pocket expenses, such as duplicating, faxing, long distance, or mileage.
5. Ask about access to the firm's law library. Such access may come in handy when the consultant needs to check on a matter related to business or the business of a client. The consultant may also want to ask whether or not the firm's conference rooms are available for the consultant's occasional use.
6. Ask about billing procedures. For example, will the consultant have 30 days within which to pay the bill? If the consultant is late in paying a bill, what interest or fees are applied?

The *Washington Business Journal* (American City Business Journals, 1993) recommends three areas of questioning in addition to those above:

1. In the event of a case against you, who will represent you?—the lawyer the consultant has interviewed, a junior partner, or a paralegal?
2. Will the consultant be an active participant in any action against him or her? Because the consultant is paying the bill, he or she should be a party to all decisions.
3. Will the consultant be kept up to date on all developments related to his or her case and supplied with ample information about the progress of the case, including documents related to the consultant and the consultant's company?

Pay attention to personal chemistry during the interview. If the attorney does not give the nurse consultant undivided attention and answers calls or constantly glances at the clock, this may not be the counsel for the nurse consultant. Look at the physical surroundings—messy or neat, cramped or spacious? Is the office equipment up to date? Look at the library. Are materials tossed helter-skelter or filed or shelved? Although it may not be easy, try to gauge the currency of the collection. Ask to see the periodicals to which the attorney or law firm subscribes. All of these clues are not only important to selection of counsel and to the counsel's currency and competency, but a gauge of the potential relationship the consultant will have down the road.

Be mindful of the consultant's rights as a client. Fallek (1991) points out that clients' rights include the following:

1. Clear answers to questions
2. Promptness, competency, and diligence in handling the consultant's work, including prompt return of calls and letters
3. Being kept up to date on work in progress
4. Fees that are reasonable and explainable
5. Itemized bill and full explanation of billing practices
6. Courtesy from all who serve the consultant
7. Uninterrupted time with counsel (object to any charges for time not completely devoted to the consultant)

These considerations for selecting legal counsel can also be applied to selecting an accountant or accounting firm, a data or information management company, a research firm, or any vendor with whom the consultant needs to work. As in any business relationship, know what is wanted from the relationship, select the vendor with care, and know and use rights accorded to the client.

Business Issues

"Prenuptial" Agreements.   Going into business with another individual or a group calls for an agreement between all parties prior to the business "marriage." The agreement should deal with the duties of all parties; the sharing in profits or losses; and buy-sell agreements as a result of the termination, loss, or death of a partner or owner. The way a business is valued is another matter for consideration prior to the consummation of a relationship with others. The name of a business may be an important matter to agree on. For example:

- Will the name of all parties to the business be the company name?
- What happens to the "ownership" of the company name on the departure of one of the owners?

- Will all parties be required to sign a noncompete agreement that prohibits each party from engaging in the same or similar business when he or she leaves the company?
- Is one or more of the owners bringing a name, trademark or patent to the business that has value that can be taken out of the business if the owner leaves?
- Do all parties have to agree to the borrowing of money or can one individual obligate the company to debt?

Insurance. "It has become a truism to say that litigation can be avoided by maintaining a good relationship with the potential litigator" (Alvarez, 1993, p. 330). Physicians are urged to improve their communication with patients to avoid malpractice suits, and many other professionals are often given the same advice about clients. The advice is applicable to the consultant as well.

In addition to communicating with clients, the consultant can also militate against potential claims of liability by having a clearly written consulting agreement. Alvarez (1993) suggests that there should be "a mechanism for evaluating the outcome of the consultation in comparison to what was contracted" (p. 330).

Still, no matter how well prepared the consultant, something can occur that results in failing to meet a standard of care, failing to fulfill a contractual obligation, or failing to meet a client's expectations. The number of suits against nurses is increasing (Scott & Beare, 1993). Thus liability insurance for the nurse consultant is important. It is important to protect the assets of the consultant in the event of a judgment against him or her. Even if the nurse consultant did nothing wrong, the cost of defending a malpractice suit can be significantly beyond most nurses' personal or business resources.

The type and amount of insurance needed will be determined by the structure of the consultant's business (e.g., a sole proprietorship or corporation) (see chapter 5). The type of consulting may influence the insurance needed. If the consultant has employees, owns or leases a car, owns or leases office space, or has sustained a previous claim or judgment, this will influence the coverage needed and the cost of coverage.

Hold Harmless Clause. Some consultants suggest the addition of a hold harmless clause to contracts with clients as one means to lessen potential liability. A hold harmless clause protects the client from any damage or injury the consultant might cause during the consultation. The consultant would be expected to compensate a client for damages from any mishaps, accidents, or bad advice. Shenson (1990) suggests that proposing a hold harmless clause may raise unnecessary anxiety in the mind of client about error or omission and may be a bad marketing strategy for the consultant.

Although a hold harmless clause is one strategy that can be combined with other mechanisms, such as insurance, it merits careful consideration with legal counsel against the backdrop of state statutes and the consultant's practice.

In the view of the authors, the best defense against malpractice is competent practice enhanced by continued learning, good communication with clients, and capable legal counsel.

Subcontracting Work. From time to time consultants will subcontract work to other consultants or receive work from other consultants. Whether the consultant is on the giving or receiving end of such work, the arrangement should be in writing. Be sure the agreement identifies clearly all work agreed to; in what form the end product is to be delivered; the due date for work to be undertaken; who is responsible for revising or refining a work product; the fees that will be paid for work done; confidentiality and copyright considerations; and a noncompete clause. A noncompete clause should preclude a subcontractor from taking the client for whom the work is done.

Vendors and Suppliers. From time to time, the consultant enters into a signed contract for goods or services. For example, the nurse consultant might lease a copier, fax, or car. The consultant might purchase a scanner or computer system with a maintenance or service agreement. All agreements with vendors or suppliers should be reviewed carefully and understood. Although many of the agreements are "boilerplate," or standardized, do not be afraid to ask questions or to ask for changes or modifications to meet unique needs. The marketplace is competitive, and this is good for the purchaser. If the vendor does not answer questions to the consultant's satisfaction or is not willing to make changes in a contract to meet the consultant's unique needs, move on. Be sure too to know the contract expiration dates or time frames in a contract that permit special buyouts or purchases.

Employees. The consultant as employer has certain legal obligations. Fallek (1991) states that employers' responsibilities fall into the areas of record keeping and standards. Record keeping entails keeping track of hours of work, wages, salaries, injuries, and illnesses. Also, employers with benefit plans, such as pension funds, will have documents to keep as well. In the area of standards, occupational safety and health requirements related to keeping the working environment safe and healthy must be met. No-smoking ordinances are one example. Other standards fall in the area of human rights, such as antidiscrimination policies and practices. Standards also must be met in the area of wages and salaries, child labor, unemployment or workers' compensation, income tax, and social security laws.

A consultant may obtain help from time to time through a temporary agency or obtain the services of a friend or family member. Care is advised in sorting through arrangements for payment; hours to be worked; the job to be done; and liability for errors, accidents, or injury.

Work Sites. Consultants just beginning to practice often work out of their homes. A number of issues that arise from working at home are addressed in chapter 5. Legal considerations also arise. A primary consideration is the consultant's liability for injury to another person or property while on the consultant's premises. For example, a customer, temporary worker or supplier might fall on the consultant's front porch or be bitten by the consultant's dog. Care must be taken to keep the home office as hazard-free as possible, and adequate insurance should be obtained to protect the consultant in the instance of injury or accident.

A work site located in a space away from one's home should also be kept hazard-free, and adequate liability insurance should be purchased. Public office space is subject to certain legal standards, which must be met. Recent laws applicable to facilities for the disabled are an example. In every instance, competent legal advice and familiarity with state and federal laws are a must.

SUMMARY

Good ethics is good business for the consultant. The ANA "Code for Nurses" and the IMC "Code of Ethics" are yardsticks to guide the consultant in day-to-day practice. Knowledge of basic legal principles, applicable laws, and good business customs; competent legal counsel; insurance protection; and generous communication with clients are safeguards for the consultant's practice.

REFERENCES

Alvarez, C. (1993). Potential liability in good consultative practice. *Clinical Nurse Specialist, 7,* 330.

American City Business Journals. (1993). Corporate counsel: How to choose a law firm. *Washington Business Journal, 12,* 49.

American Nurses Association. (1976). *Code for nurses with interpretive statements.* Kansas City: Author.

Churchill, L. (1977). Ethical issues of a profession in transition. *American Journal of Nursing, 77,* 873.

Cohen, W. (1991). *How to make it big as a consultant.* New York: AMACOM.

Fallek, M. (1991). *How to set up your own small business.* Minneapolis: American Institute of Small Business.

Guttenberg, J. (1995). Good reputation may be a firm's biggest asset. *Washington Business Journal, 14,* 27.

Holtz, H. (1993). *How to succeed as an independent consultant* (3rd ed.). New York: John Wiley & Sons.

Institute of Management Consultants. (1991). *Code of ethics.* New York: Council of Consulting Organizations.

Martindale-Hubbell Law Directory. (1995). Chicago: R.R. Donnelley & Sons.

Scott, L., & Beare, P. (1993). Nurse consultant and professional liability. *Clinical Nurse Specialist, 7,* 331.

Shenson, H. (1990). *On consulting.* New York: Wiley with University Associates.

Ulschak, F. L., & SnowAntle, S. M. (1990). *Consultation skills for health care professionals.* San Francisco: Jossey-Bass.

Weiss, A. (1992). *Million dollar consulting: The professional's guide to growing a practice.* New York: McGraw-Hill.

9

The Consultant as a Person

The nurse consultant will find that the work consumes a great deal of time, particularly in the first stages of starting a consulting practice. The hard work does not lessen, however, as the roster of clients grows and marketing efforts continue. One of the downsides that may occur with a successful business is that the consultant finds himself or herself with no life other than work. To avoid that, in this chapter some ways of getting and staying organized, managing time, and otherwise creating a life away from work are presented.

A caveat is necessary here: Consulting is a business characterized by "peaks and valleys." There are times when the nurse consultant may be frenetically busy and other times when it seems as if the telephone will *never* ring. Recognizing that these periods of feast or famine, or flood and drought, occur is the first step in dealing with them. The nurse consultant who devotes time to marketing on an ongoing basis (see chapter 6) is less likely to experience periods of severe drought.

It is important when slack periods occur not to give up and decide that consulting is not all it promised to be. The nurse consultant who thinks that "if this doesn't work out, I can always go back to the hospital" is not likely to be a success at consulting, because he or she is not totally committed.

Although this chapter is primarily targeted toward nurse consultants in their own businesses, the strategies offered are also applicable to the internal nurse consultant or intrepreneur in the health care setting (see chapter 4).

GETTING ORGANIZED

Being organized is a hallmark of an efficient individual. Efficiency, in turn, can lead to effectiveness. Because most nurse consultants work alone, it is essential for them to be efficient as well as effective in their work.

Time is a valuable commodity for the nurse consultant, as for anyone else. Moreover, the nurse consultant relies on billable time for his or her livelihood, so it is imperative that time be spent as expeditiously as possible.

Getting organized in one's environment as well as in one's work habits will save time—time that might better be devoted to other work-related activities. Lack of organization is an insidious stealer of time. Ten years ago, Booher (1986) noted that "Studies of American business indicate that 50 to 70 percent of all working hours are spent on paperwork" (p. 2). Imagine the increase in that figure that must have occurred over the last decade!

Booher cites other frightening statistics, including the following:

Three percent of needed documents are misfiled.
Seventy-five percent to 85% of all documents filed are never referred to again.

The costs of such waste and inefficiency are staggering.

Nurse consultants deal with paperwork, just as do clerical, managerial, and white-collar workers in industry. In a nurse consultant's files can be found proposals, reports of projects, correspondence, budgets, and many other documents that may create needless paperwork and increase the cost of doing business as well as keep the individual from more pleasurable pursuits.

Handling Mail

A variety of ways exist to manage paperwork. One of the most successful is to handle a piece of paper only once. Incoming mail is a good example. The nurse consultant would open each piece of mail and decide immediately what to do with it, according to the 4-D system (Livesay, 1994, pp. 36–37):

1. Don't open it.
2. Discard it.
3. Designate it for action.
4. Direct it.

Incoming mail should be opened near a wastebasket, so that "junk" mail and mail that is to be discarded immediately after it is opened can be disposed of right away. The danger in not tossing mail immediately is that it clutters a desktop or other working surfaces for some time before finally being discarded.

Mail on which action needs to be taken can be immediately filed in a file folder located where the mail is opened. Thus, invoices can be placed in a

"Bills to Be Paid" file until checks are written; correspondence can be filed until a time when the nurse consultant can answer it all at once, thus taking advantage of the momentum that occurs in writing to facilitate responses.

The nurse consultant working alone may not have anyone in his or her business to whom to direct mail. In this case, the nurse consultant may route the information to someone outside of the business who might be interested in the contents of the mail. This is an effective strategy to keep in touch with current as well as prospective clients.

Organizing Files

A great deal of information resides in an individual's files; Booher (1986) states that the annual cost of maintaining an "active four-drawer file of 18,000 pages" is $2,160. Some strategies for organizing files include saving only those materials to which the nurse consultant would not otherwise have access (e.g., at a library or from a client or colleague); saving only one copy of any material; putting a destruction date on every piece of paper, after which it is discarded; and purging files at least once a year.

Color coding files helps organize them. A different color can be assigned to each project, or to a certain type of file: for example, blue for contracts and red for progress reports.

Keeping files as thin as possible also helps in storage and retrieval. Individuals with "fat" files expend effort on leafing through a file to find a particular item; the item stored by itself in a thin file would be more easily retrievable.

Tuller (1992) recommends the personal computer as a way of managing the large amount of paper associated with consulting work. Software programs can handle some consulting tasks, such as writing reports, invoicing, keeping track of hours expended and expenses incurred; and the information generated during these activities can be stored on the computer (on the hard drive or on diskettes) as well.

Dealing with paperwork is only a part of getting organized, but admittedly it is a big part!

A Six-Step Process for Getting Organized

General advice for getting organized is offered by Livesay (1994), as a six-step process:

1. Deciding what should be organized
2. Getting rid of clutter
3. Breaking organizing tasks into specific steps
4. Establishing a simple system

5. Staying organized
6. Being only as organized as necessary

Deciding What Should Be Organized. Livesay (1994) uses the 80/20 rule—also referred to as the Pareto principle—to help decide what should be organized in an individual's life. The 80/20 rule states that 80% of anything of value comes from only 20% of effort. Examples of the 80/20 rule in networking are that 80% of referrals, business opportunities, and other benefits result from 20% of an individual's contacts (see chapter 7); in a retail business, 80% of sales come from 20% of the products.

In the nurse consultant's business, the first step is to decide what are the high-payoff areas—that is, the 20% that will result in 80% of the value of getting organized. An assessment of the work environment and work activities will help determine the high-payoff areas. For example, the consultant may need to have the area around his or her telephone organized, whereas the top of the desk does not need to be organized—or vice versa. Some filing cabinet drawers must be organized because items in those drawers are referred to frequently, whereas other drawers are not as essential because information in those drawers is accessed infrequently. Livesay suggests that the high-payoff areas are those that are used frequently in a day, contribute substantially to the ability to perform a work activity, and are an integral part of the flow of the work to be done.

Uncluttering Life. Getting rid of clutter is essential to getting organized. Clutter accumulates when people save everything, thinking there will be a use for it later. Overstuffed filing cabinets are a good example of the results of this "pack rat" behavior. Individuals who tend to procrastinate also tend to accumulate clutter because they cannot make a decision about what to do about something—a memo, for example. Should it be filed, routed, or responded to? Since the decision is not made, the memo is generally placed on a desktop or in a filing cabinet and then is seen no more.

To deal with clutter, Livesay suggests that individuals set limits on what they own—two filing cabinets, for instance. When those two cabinets are full, materials are thrown away rather than purchasing—and filling—another filing cabinet. Keeping articles of interest rather than complete issues of journals will reduce clutter. If something has not been used for a given time—a year, for example—it should be discarded. This principle has been used with some success by one of the authors: Periodically, everything on the desk or tabletop is swept into an empty drawer. The drawer is sealed with tape on which a date—usually 4 to 6 months later—is written. If the drawer has not been raided to seek information of vital importance during the specified time, on the date written on the tape the drawer is opened, and everything in the drawer is discarded. It is vital not to look at anything as it is being thrown away; otherwise, it will be saved—just in case. It may even be necessary to have someone else open the drawer and discard the contents, to avoid peeking.

This method also works with business cards. It is necessary to purge a Rolodex periodically because the 80/20 rule applies here as well. It can safely be assumed that 80 percent of business cards that are saved will not be referred to again. Ensign (1991) recommends thinning out the Rolodex while on hold, placing a paper clip on the card last reviewed. Another way is to rubber-band a stack of business cards and place them in the drawer with a date noted on the top of the stack. If by the date noted the stack has not been rifled to find an individual's card, the entire stack can be discarded.

Breaking Organizational Tasks into Specific Steps. Procrastination often occurs when an individual is faced with a major project. The project seems overwhelming, and thus is put off again and again, while time that could be spent on it is wasted on minutiae. One way to overcome procrastination is to "just do it," but this may be difficult. It often is easier to attack only one part of the project at a time.

In an instance where the project is evaluation of the effectiveness of a statewide system of continuing education, for example, the nurse consultant might use a "backward" system of setting goals for completion of project activities as follows:

December—final report due
November—draft report written
October—data analysis completed
September—data collection finished
August—data collection started
July—interim progress report due
June—data collection sources identified
May—data collection methods developed
April—data collection methods approved
March—data collection methods suggested
February—project goals and objectives approved
January—project goals and objectives identified

Thus, the project now appears to be a series of small steps, each of which can be accomplished in a reasonable time frame, rather than an overwhelming year-long project. It is also likely that the nurse consultant will accomplish more on the project than just the one step identified for each month. The momentum that follows just getting started may propel the nurse consultant forward into the next month's activity even before it is due to be started.

It is important to set up a reward system for accomplishing an activity. The reward can be going out to lunch, purchasing a new piece of clothing, or taking an afternoon off to see a movie. The reward does not need to be large; its purpose is serve as motivation to complete the activity.

Establishing a Simple System.   Some systems that purport to help people become organized require a great deal of organization themselves. Livesay suggests that systems must not require a great deal of maintenance; items must be placed within convenient reach; and materials for projects should be all kept in one place.

One simple system is to view a desktop as a workplace rather than a storage place. Only work to be accomplished may be on the desk. All materials not related to the work at hand are stored elsewhere. Then, when a project is to be addressed, all relevant files and other materials are moved to the desktop, but nothing not related to the project appears on the desk top to serve as a source of distraction. When work on one project has been completed, the project materials are moved elsewhere for storage and the materials for the next project are brought to the desktop. This method has the added benefit of keeping stacks of papers off the desk and thus reducing clutter. Livesay asserts that "Executives spend an average of 30 minutes a day (or a full workday per month) searching desktop piles for papers" (p. 69). Using the desktop as a work area rather than as a storage area should reduce or eliminate this time-waster.

Staying Organized.   Once a system has been established and implemented, and is working, it should be kept in place. It is more difficult to get organized again once things start to slide than it is to maintain a system. A few new skills may be all that is necessary to maintain a system; one of the most important of these skills is to develop the habit of putting everything in its place so that valuable time is not spent searching for something.

Being Only as Organized as Necessary.   Caution must be exercised so that getting organized does not become an end in itself rather than a means to an end. There always will be someone more organized, so striving for perfection in organization is not an effective use of time or energy. The goal should be to be only as organized as necessary to accomplish the work that needs to be done with the greatest level of efficiency and effectiveness. For example, it may not be necessary to have an elaborate color-coded, alphabetized filing system if the nurse consultant is the only one using it. If the nurse consultant sees clients at his or her office, however, the work space should appear organized and uncluttered.

Whatever system is used for getting organized, it is important to adapt it to the nurse consultant's work habits and environment. Rarely can a system be adopted in its entirety; to prevent frustration, it is crucial to know what will work in the situation and what will not.

Getting organized and staying organized are two skills that nurse consultants need in order to accomplish their work. The time spent on getting organized initially and maintaining that level of organization will pay off handsomely. Once a satisfactory level of organization is achieved, the nurse consultant will be ready to devote some energy to making the best use of his or her time.

MANAGING TIME

To manage time effectively, the first step is to identify the activities to which time is currently devoted. Thus, it is necessary to keep a time log on which daily activity is noted in 15-minute increments for at least a week. All activities should be logged, even those not directly related to work, such as travel to clients' locations, filing, eating meals, and personal activities, such as reading or watching television. The totals for all of these activities should be calculated.

This log is helpful in identifying the use of time, but also can be used to track hours devoted to specific projects. A time log can provide data to substantiate the time necessary to devote to certain projects and to calculate the nurse consultant's billable hours (see chapter 5).

Mancini (1994) suggests that the totals on the time log be reviewed to answer the following questions:

- What is the activity that consumes the most time?
- What is the activity that consumes the second most time?
- What activities constitute the greatest work time?
- What activities constitute the greatest personal time?
- What are the time-consuming non-work-related activities?
- Are there any time-consuming activities that are a surprise?
- On what activities should more time be spent?
- On what activities should less time be spent?

This review should provide an indication of current use of time. Then, the nurse consultant can use what was learned to manage time more effectively—emphasizing the areas on which more time needs to be spent, and seeking ways to minimize time spent in nonproductive activities. It may be that one hour less of watching television a week, for instance, will allow the nurse consultant to catch up on his or her reading, or attending one less weekly meeting of a social group a month will permit time to be spent in organizing the work space, thus leading to greater productivity.

Lack of time management often leads to stress. The individual feels that things are out of control and that he or she cannot manage everything that needs to be done. Actually, most of this stress is generated by the individual and can be avoided by using effective time management techniques both at work and in his or her personal life. Effectively managing time at work means that time can be allocated to personal activities that might otherwise not be considered because of perceived workload.

Making Lists and Setting Priorities

One of the most effective time management techniques is to make lists of what is to be accomplished. Winston (1995) suggests that a master list be kept, on which everything is written down as soon as it is comes to mind. A spiral notebook kept in the same place on the desk at all times is a good place to do this recording. The notebook also can be used to track telephone conversations, providing a reliable memory aid.

Items that must be done then can be transferred to another daily list, a "to do" reminder. Priorities should be set, using the A-B-C system, where A is a "must do today" item; B is "important but not critical," and C can be done if time permits. Attention should be devoted to the A tasks first— and only when these are completed should energy be focused on the B and C tasks. As activities are completed, they should be crossed off the list. Items that have not been accomplished by the end of the day can be transferred to the next day's list.

Items to be accomplished can be written on "post-it" notes or small scraps of paper and placed on a clipboard or bulletin board and discarded as each is finished. Getting rid of the reminder of the task (crossing it off a list; throwing away a post-it note) is satisfying and may help motivate the nurse consultant to proceed with another task.

Mancini (1994) recommends setting up a filing system, where letter trays are labeled A, B, and C. Items related to the priorities labeled with these letters then are filed in the appropriate tray. Items are moved up or downward depending on the priority assigned to them, which may change over time (as items with an A designation are completed, some B items may assume more urgency and thus deserve A status). Once each week, all items stored in the C tray are reviewed. It may be that the status of these items has changed to the extent that some do not need to be accomplished at all.

An electronic system of scheduling tasks can be used; there are a number of software packages for this purpose. One system (Microsoft Scheduler) displays preset daily planner pages on which the user can enter tasks for specific time periods. A visible reminder of each task then pops up on the screen at the appointed time; this is accompanied by an audible signal in case the user is not working at the computer when a reminder is flashed. The program allows the user to delay notification again for a specific time or to turn off notification. Appointments can be moved to another time, day, month, or year; the program contains a perpetual calendar. Appointments can be deleted as they are accomplished. And the program allows for a daily schedule to be printed for a visual overview of the entire day.

Winston (1995), however, suggests that rather than focus first on the most important tasks (the As) each day, the individual should strive to complete a variety of tasks each day, selecting from among the A, B, and C priorities. In that way, she holds the demands on an individual will be lessened because some tasks will not require as much concentration, and these tasks can be accomplished during low-energy times, such as after lunch.

Ensign (1991) suggests that a time limit be set for each activity on a "to do" list and that this time limit not be exceeded. She also recommends that an individual be cognizant of his or her peak working time and devote that time to major projects, spending nonpeak working time doing "low-brain" activities, such as organizing, filing, or reading.

Hedrick (1990) suggests a different strategy for a "to do" list: The individual notes not only "external" appointments, such as meetings, sessions with clients, or lunch engagements; but also "internal" appointments, those that the individual makes with himself or herself, such as the decision to complete a progress report by a certain date. This method leads to treatment of internal appointments and external appointments as equally important.

Overcoming Procrastination

Mancini (1994) asserts that procrastination is the worst time-waster. He suggests a number of strategies to overcome what may appear to be a difficult habit to break:

1. Do an unpleasant task first thing in the morning—once it is out of the way, the relief will be motivating.
2. Change routines, such as the route taken to an appointment—a different way of doing things will break down barriers.
3. Do nothing—simply sit in the office and stare out the window. Boredom will soon take hold, and working will seem easier.
4. Cluster tasks, such as answering correspondence—the momentum of making telephone calls or writing letters will often increase productivity significantly.
5. Take advantage of the chronological clock in each individual that controls energy output—schedule difficult tasks during peak times;

avoid doing any one task for more than 1½ hours; and eat lean protein meals at lunch.
6. Delegate any task that can possibly be delegated.

Delegating Work

Mancini (1994) also describes 12 steps of "masterful delegation":

1. Identify the task to be delegated.
2. Specify the way the task should be completed.
3. Find the right person to whom to delegate the task.
4. Explain the task.
5. Explain the benefits of the individual's completing the task.
6. Specify the standards for completion.
7. Present deadlines.
8. Establish a method for reporting progress.
9. Ask for questions.
10. Check on progress periodically.
11. Assess results.
12. Recognize achievement.

It may be difficult for the nurse consultant to consider delegating tasks to others; but thinking that they can better be accomplished by himself or herself, often is a fallacy. Most tasks that are not critical priorities can be accomplished by someone else with the same effectiveness. It may help for the nurse consultant to think about the cost of his or her doing the task versus paying someone else to do the same task. Thus, the consultant can compare the loss of 1 billable hour at $200 with paying someone perhaps $10 to accomplish the same task.

Another strategy is to adopt the principle of "satisficing," that is: What will satisfy the requirements? Many women, for example, do not wish to employ a housekeeper because someone else might not clean house as well as they would; yet if the housekeeper can meet standards that "satisfy" the employer, extra time will result to devote to other activities. Likewise, in business, the nurse consultant may be satisfied with having someone else make photocopies, file, or open mail, deciding that the other individual's system for doing so may not be the system he or she would use, but that it satisfies the requirements for making photocopies, filing, or opening mail.

Avoiding Time-Wasters

Other useful tips offered by Mancini (1994) relate to use of the telephone to avoid wasting time. Some of these tips follow:

- Minimize introductory remarks—go straight to the point of the call.
- Make notes of what should be covered on a call in advance of making the call.
- Keep track of the time spent on a call; if the telephone does not have a built-in timer, use an egg timer. This strategy will help minimize the cost of long-distance calls.
- Take notes of every telephone call; use the spiral notebook mentioned earlier to track what was agreed on during the call and what follow-up action, if any, is needed.
- Use a speaker telephone or a headset to avoid having to hold the receiver while on hold; use time on hold for other activities, such as thinning a Rolodex or straightening a desk.
- Use automatic redial to deal with a busy signal.
- To avoid "telephone tag," make an appointment to return a call if the person is not available at the time the initial call is placed.
- If the individual being called is on another line, ask to be placed on hold and use the waiting time to accomplish other tasks.
- Leave messages that contain a specific time when a return call would be convenient; let the caller know what is expected on a return call so that he or she can be prepared.
- Note the sequence numbers ("to reach Personnel, press 1; for Administration, press 2") for automated telephone systems that are frequently used, so time is not wasted listening to the entire message.

Another strategy that may help the nurse consultant deal with time-wasters is to learn to say "no." Unfortunately, this is probably the most difficult technique to learn and to practice. One strategy that may make saying no more acceptable to the nurse consultant is to give a reason. The reason should be offered calmly and firmly. Sometimes it is easier to decline if the "no" is "sandwiched" between other statements, such as "I really would like to help with the project, but I can't at this time, because I am overloaded right now." Any attempt to overcome saying no should be met with repetition of the statement.

It is important to be tactful and kind when declining something; sandwiching the refusal between two "nice" statements makes it easier to say and perhaps easier to hear as well. Offering to make a trade also may work: In this case, the nurse consultant declines one activity (serving as chair of a conference planning committee) but offers to serve as a moderator at the conference, for example. Alternatively, the nurse consultant can offer to be involved in the same activity at a future date.

One strategy that should *not* be used is to offer to "think it over" before making a commitment. This is a form of procrastination and is unfair to the requester, because it simply delays the decision.

What may not be needed to manage time is the latest gadget being touted as a time-saver. It is important to assess both the advantages and disadvantages of timesaving systems. Although many items do save time (the fax, for example), others—such as elaborate calendars, preprinted "to do" lists, and even some software packages—may be unnecessary or may require so much time to learn that they defeat the original purpose.

MANAGING WORK AND HOME

Although the demands of work may be heavy, it is important for the nurse consultant to seek to balance those demands with others, such as those imposed by family and the community. At the outset, it is crucial to determine what the nurse consultant perceives as important for a satisfying life. It may be that working provides a great deal of satisfaction, while devoting time to community activities seems more a burden than a pleasure. Family may take priority while children are young, but when they are older and off to school and the spouse is working as well, the nurse consultant may find it pleasurable to devote most of his or her time to work-related activities.

MANAGING STRESS

Inability to balance the demands of life often causes stress that affects the individual physically and psychologically and affects both work and home life. Change is a notorious stress producer, yet change is occurring more rapidly than ever before: Witness the explosion in technology that shows no signs of stopping, or even slowing down. It is impossible to maintain the status quo, so it is incumbent on the nurse consultant to learn to manage stress.

Tips for Stress Management

Some tips for stress management have been offered by Badger (1995):

- Begin to breathe deeply as soon as the feeling of being stressed becomes apparent.
- If possible, do some stretching exercises—rolling the neck from side to center to side is relaxing, as is moving the shoulders toward the ears in a shrug, then relaxing them.
- Assess immediate priorities. Some of the activities that are creating stress can be postponed; try to accomplish only those activities that are urgent and defer the others until a less stressful time.

- Focus on what has been done rather than on what remains to be done.
- Set realistic expectations—always allot much more time than anticipated to a task, and start it well before the deadline for completion.
- Take breaks, and eat meals.
- Review situations that cause stress to determine what could be done in the future to avoid it or handle it better.

Factors in Stress Management

Galginaitis (1994) offers some useful advice about managing stress by managing the demands of work and home. She suggests that individuals identify factors in their lives over which they have control and those outside their sphere of influence, and then concentrate on changing what needs to be changed within the individual's sphere of influence, because those factors over which the individual has no control are not likely to be changed by his or her efforts. Thus, the individual can seek to eliminate the source of stress, change perceptions of stress, or avoid situations that cause stress.

Among the other suggestions offered by Galginaitis (1994) are to

- Promote emotional health.
- Promote physical health.
- Manage time effectively.
- Minimize household responsibilities.
- Review other commitments.
- Eliminate job stress.
- Consider a job change.

Each of these factors will be considered in some detail below.

Promote Emotional Health.   An individual who is not emotionally healthy will not be able to withstand the rigors of work, with its attendant stress, nor will that individual be able to balance the demands of work and home life. To achieve what is desired, the nurse consultant should set priorities to identify activities that are really important; maintain reasonable expectations for himself or herself and others; ask for help when needed; and stay flexible and adaptable to change.

Promote Physical Health.   Individuals who are not physically fit generally are more stressed. Exercising regularly is a proven way of increasing energy and reducing stress. A busy nurse consultant may not have the time to devote to long periods of exercise, however, so increased activity throughout the day may have to substitute. Climbing stairs rather than riding elevators, parking in the back of a parking lot and walking to the mall, and similar activities can increase the amount of daily exercise. Nothing, however, will really replace for a planned exercise regimen.

Eating a healthy diet is important. Also, some evidence now exists that taking a 20-minute nap in the afternoon is healthy, as it both relaxes and energizes individuals. Proponents suggest not taking the nap after 4:00 P.M., however, as the nap might then interfere with a good night's sleep. It is also important to turn off the telephone and fax—and not to feel guilty. Taking time out for activities other than work also will promote both physical and emotional health.

Manage Time Effectively. The nurse constant must learn to use time advantageously, taking advantage of any tactics that seem to work for others. For example, both authors purchase greeting cards once a year for all occasions. They takes a list of special occasions (birthdays, weddings, and anniversaries) and select cards with specific people in mind. In addition, they purchase a great stack of "generic" cards—"Thank You," "Get Well," "Congratulations," and "Happy Birthday"—to use all year long. This saves a great deal of time, which would otherwise be spent in individual trips to the card store.

Another timesaving strategy is to shop by mail for holiday and birthday gifts. Avoiding crowded malls not only saves time but it reduces stress. Another shopping strategy is to purchase Christmas gifts all year long— whenever something is spotted that would make a nice gift for someone. These gifts are stored in one place in the house, so they can easily be retrieved and cataloged well before the holiday. In addition to making gift purchasing easier, this technique also spreads the cost over an entire year.

Shopping while traveling for meetings and conferences—for instance, when there is "down time"—anyway saves time for more important activities at home. Purchases made away from home can be shipped at little cost to avoid having to carry them.

Minimize Household Responsibilities. Whenever possible, hire people to get housework done. Teenagers can mow lawns, rake leaves, and shovel snow. They also can be employed at reasonable rates to watch children for an afternoon, make copies, prepare a mailing, and perform other tasks that free the nurse consultant to do the work only he or she can do. Often area high schools have work-study programs where students are encouraged to work as part of their learning experiences; these teens generally are willing workers and do not require large salaries.

Hiring outside help may make it necessary to lower expectations for how these delegated tasks are to be accomplished—it may mean that the house is cleaned less thoroughly, for example, or less frequently. Galginaitis (1994) suggests some creative ways of managing to do more with less: holding a "cook-in" where neighbors all cook meals that can be frozen and reheated for dinners, perhaps trading meals for variety; cooking large batches of favorite dishes, serving one recipe, and freezing the rest for later, and bartering services, such as child care or housecleaning for lawn care.

Review Other Commitments. It is generally not possible to devote equal amounts of energy to a variety of commitments, so it is necessary to ascertain those which are most important to the individual. One way of doing this is to list all current commitments and rank them according to the amount of energy they require in comparison with the value received. Then activities on the bottom of the list—those that require a great deal of energy for little payoff—can be eliminated or severely curtailed.

Eliminate Job Stress. The nurse consultant should periodically review work commitments, both current and future, with a critical eye. Sometimes, it is wise to say "no" to new business, even if it means additional income, if the new project will add unneeded stress. Although this may be difficult to do, declining a project generally will lead not to loss of business but to the perception that the nurse consultant is in demand and worth the price of his or her services. Several years ago a well-known consultant revealed that she had too much business and sought to reduce her workload by increasing her fee rather than saying "no," so she doubled her fee. Strangely enough, the increase did not deter clients, so she was left with no recourse other than saying "no."

Consider a Job Change. Consultation is a job, just as is a position with an employer. It may be necessary for the consultant to review his or her workload, and pare it down to reasonable proportions. Simply removing those parts of the job that are not satisfying or difficult may suffice, but it may also be necessary to eliminate portions of an activity, or the activity itself. For example, the nurse consultant who conducts outcome research may have difficulty with statistical analysis of the data he or she has collected, and may decide that it would be less stressful and much more efficient to outsource the data analysis portion of the project to a local university. The nurse consultant may also be working with a child with special education needs in the home and having difficulty obtaining the cooperation of the parents. In that case, it may be wise for the nurse consultant to refer the client to another resource rather than continue to create the same stress for himself or herself.

Stress Management and Family

Nurse consultants with spouses and children have special demands on their time. Galginaitis (1994) offers some good advice about relationships with spouse and children:

- Take time for the spouse.
- Share household tasks.
- Plan time with children.
- Obtain necessary child care.

With family and friends, it is important for consultants to do the following:

- Formulate plans for care of elderly parents.
- Spend time with parents.
- Spend time with friends.
- Ask for support.

As can been seen, Galginaitis places emphasis on relationships that serve to provide meaning to individuals' lives. Although work may produce a great deal of satisfaction for the nurse consultant, relationships with spouse, children, family, and friends also play a key role in a well-balanced and, thus, productive and satisfying lifestyle.

SUMMARY

In this chapter, some ideas for getting and staying organized and managing time were offered. Many other tips can be suggested for balancing the demands of work and home. It is important mainly to be clear about what needs to be accomplished, and which of those things that must be done are important enough to warrant the nurse consultant's time and energy. Clear and specific goals make the task easier. If the nurse consultant has an idea of where he or she wants to go in professional and personal life, activities that do not contribute to this vision will not be undertaken. But activities that do enhance the possibility that professional and personal goals will be accomplished will be undertaken, because accomplishing them will move the consultant toward his or her career goals and contribute to a feeling of satisfaction.

REFERENCES

Badger, J. M. (1995). 14 tips for managing stress on the job. *American Journal of Nursing, 95,* 31–33.

Booher, D. (1986). *Cutting paperwork in the corporate culture.* New York: Facts on File.

Ensign, P. (1991). *110 ideas for organizing your business life.* Bedford Hills, NY: Organizing Solutions.

Galginaitis, C. R. (1994). *Managing the demands of work and home.* Burr Ridge, IL: Irwin.

Hedrick, L. H. (1990). *Five days to an organized life.* New York: Dell.

Livesay, C. R. (1994). *Getting and staying organized.* Burr Ridge, IL: Irwin.

Mancini, M. (1994). *Time management.* Burr Ridge, IL: Irwin.

Tuller, L. W. (1992). *The independent consultant's Q&A book.* Holbrook, MA: Bob Adams.

Winston, S. (1995). *Stephanie Winston's best organizing tips.* New York: Simon & Schuster.

Appendix: Resources

Small Business Administration
409 Third Street SW
Washington, DC 20416

Small Business Investment Companies
409 Third Street SW
Washington, DC 20416

National Association of Female Executives
30 Irving Place, 5th Floor
New York, NY 10003

National Nurses in Business Association
1000 Burnett Avenue
Suite 450
Concord, CA 94520

National Association of Women Business Owners
1413 K Street, Northwest, Suite 637
Washington, DC 20005

Index

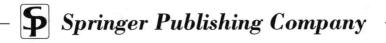

Springer Publishing Company

INCREASING PATIENT SATISFACTION
A Guide for Nurses

Roberta L. Messner, RNC, PhD, CPHQ
Susan J. Lewis, RN, PhD, CS

This manual guides nurses and others in the health care setting through the fundamentals of ensuring a satisfied "customer." It illustrates the many components of quality care, including how to provide clear and adequate information, create a hospitable environment, handle complaints efficiently, and design and utilize surveys of client satisfaction.

The authors draw from the principles of continuous quality improvement and other lessons learned from the business world, in addition to nursing's rich tradition of service. Written with warmth, sensitivity, and clarity, the book is an excellent resource for nursing students and practicing nurses. Health care institutions seeking good client relations will find this a suitable text for in-service training.

Contents:

What Do Patients Really Want? • The Changing American Healthcare Scene and Patient Satisfaction• Quality Isn't a Coincidence• Yes, Patients Do Have Rights • Patient Education: A Key to Increased Satisfaction • Creating a Hospitable and Healing Environment • How to Handle a Customer Complaint • Looking for the Lesson: Measuring/Evaluating Patient Satisfaction Findings • Be Kind to Yourself and Your Coworkers: A Plan for Enhanced Morale and Patient Satisfaction

1996   240pp   0-8261-9250-5   hardcover

536 Broadway, New York, NY 10012-3955 • (212) 431-4370 • Fax (212) 941-7842

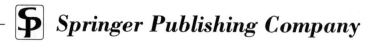
Springer Publishing Company

SUCCESSFUL GRANT WRITING
Strategies for Health and Human Service Professionals

Laura N. Gitlin, PhD and **Kevin J. Lyons,** PhD

This book guides the reader through the language and basic components of grantmanship. It illustrates how to develop ideas for funding, write the sections of a proposal, organize different types of project structures, and finally, how to understand the review process.

Each chapter describes a specific aspect of grantmanship and suggests innovative strategies to implement the information that is presented. The appendices contain helpful materials, such as a list of key acronyms, examples of timelines and sample budget sheets. The strategies in this volume are beneficial to individuals and departments in academic, clinical, or community-based settings.

> SUCCESSFUL
> GRANT
> WRITING
> *Strategies for Health and Human Service Professionals*
>
> LAURA N. GITLIN. PHD
> KEVIN J. LYONS. PHD
>
> **$**
> *Springer Publishing Company*

Partial Contents:
- Becoming Familiar with Funding Sources
- Developing Your Ideas for Funding
- Learning about Your Institution
- Common Sections of Proposals
- Preparing a Budget
- Technical Considerations
- Strategies for Effective Writing
- Understanding the Process of Collaboration
- Understanding the Review Process

1996   235pp   0-8261-9260-2   hard cover

536 Broadway, New York, NY 10012-3955 • (212) 431-4370 • Fax (212) 941-7842

Springer Publishing Company

Developing a Private Practice in Psychiatric Mental-Health Nursing
Susanne Fine, MA, RN, CS

This book is a how-to manual for managing the business aspects of a private practice in psychiatric mental health nursing. The author shares the practical information earned from long experience in private practice, including the legal requirements for practice, how to start up a practice and market your services, how to explain what a nurse psychotherapist is to those who don't know, methods for recordkeeping and billing, fee schedules, and negotiating third-party reimbursement including managed care. This book includes over twenty useful sample forms and letters (i.e. a sample letter for denial of insurance claims). It also includes a listing of insurance companies and managed care companies, with addresses.

Developing a Private Practice in Psychiatric Mental-Health Nursing

Susanne Fine

The book concludes with a comprehensive state-by-state summary of educational and practice requirements for advanced practice nurses. Nurses embarking on a career in advanced practice mental health will find this manual invaluable. It can also be useful to other mental-health practitioners, since many of the same reimbursement and practice issues are relevant.

Springer Series on Advanced Practice Nursing
1997   184pp   0-8261-9440-0   hardcover

536 Broadway, New York, NY 10012-3955 • (212) 431-4370 • Fax (212) 941-7842

$\boxed{\text{SP}}$ *Springer Publishing Company*

ANNUAL REVIEW OF NURSING RESEARCH
Volume 14: Focus on Nursing Intervention

Joyce J. Fitzpatrick, PhD
Jane Norbeck, DNSc, *Editors*

This landmark series draws together and critically reviews all the
existing research in specific areas of
nursing practice, nursing care delivery, nursing education, and the
profession of nursing.

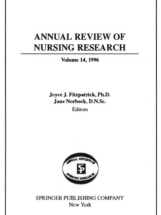

**ANNUAL REVIEW OF
NURSING RESEARCH**

Volume 14, 1996

Joyce J. Fitzpatrick, Ph.D.
Jane Norbeck, D.N.Sc.
Editors

SPRINGER PUBLISHING COMPANY
New York

Contents:

- Blood Pressure
- Psychoneuroimmunological
  Studies in HIV Disease
- Delirium Intervention Research
  in Acute Care Settings
- Smoking Cessation Interventions
  in Chronic Illness
- Quality of Life and Caregiving in Technological Home Care
- Organizational Redesign: Effects on Institutional
  and Consumer Outcomes
- Organizational Culture
- Oncology Nursing Education
- Moral Competency
- Nursing Research in Israel
- The Evolution of Nursing Research in Brazil

1996   280pp   0-8261-8233-X   hardcover

536 Broadway, New York, NY 10012-3955 • (212) 431-4370 • Fax (212) 941-7842